Now This In  *dispensable Volume*
Offers Up
Infor

- **Postpartum blues,** compassionate advice from other mothers

- **Breast-feeding vs. bottle-feeding**—the latest information on feeding schedules

- **Fathering**—new findings on father-infant attachment

- **Preventing SIDS**—the sleeping position recommended for your infant's safety

- **Weaning**—helpful hints on when to begin, and how to wean to a bottle or a cup

- **Introducing solid foods**—guidelines to aid in starting your baby on solids

- **Swimming lessons**—when and how to start, and why it's such a good idea

- **Formation of teeth**—dealing with crankiness, diarrhea, and dental care

- Plus the latest advice for **working mothers** and new findings on **cesarean births, infant sleep schedules, selecting commercially prepared baby foods,** and much more.

The

First Twelve
Months of Life

YOUR BABY'S
GROWTH
MONTH BY MONTH

The Princeton Center for Infancy
and Early Childhood

Frank Caplan, Founder ● Theresa Caplan, Director

BANTAM BOOKS
NEW YORK • TORONTO • LONDON • SYDNEY • AUCKLAND

CODMAN SQUARE

This edition contains the complete text
of the original hardcover edition.
NOT ONE WORD HAS BEEN OMITTED.

THE FIRST TWELVE MONTHS OF LIFE
A Bantam Book / published in association
with the Putnam Publishing Group

PUBLISHING HISTORY
Perigree Books edition published 1993
Bantam edition / July 1995

ISBN 0-553-57406-X

Published simultaneously in the United States and Canada

PRINTED IN THE UNITED STATES OF AMERICA

OPM   0   9   8   7   6

This revised and updated
edition is dedicated to
the loving memory of Frank Caplan
June 10, 1911–September 28, 1988
and
mothers and fathers and
their babies everywhere.

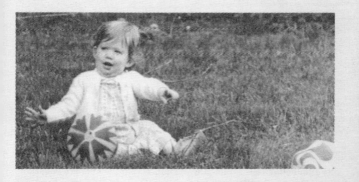

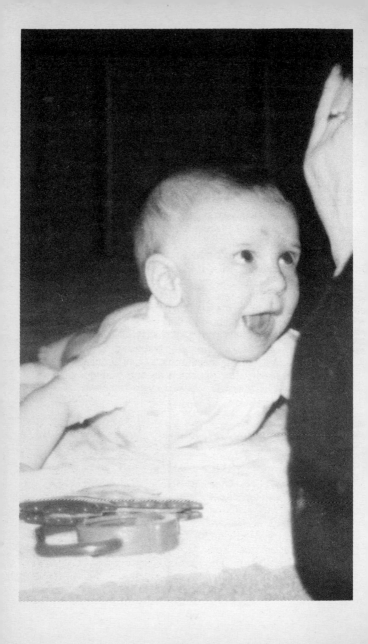

Acknowledgments

This book exists because of the cooperation, encouragement, and information supplied by many researchers working with infants and their mothers and fathers, and the diligence of a staff who for two years painstakingly put together the accumulated bits and pieces of pertinent data into a readable manuscript.

We especially wish to thank Dr. T. Berry Brazelton, eminent pediatrician and research fellow at Harvard's Center for Cognitive Studies. Many of the ideas in this revised and updated book have been inspired by Dr. Brazelton's fine work, *Infants and Mothers: Differences in Development*. However, he is not responsible for any of the ideas or judgments expressed herein, unless directly attributed to him.

We are also grateful to the many outstanding professional infancy and parenting researchers and educators who shared their fascinating experiences and findings with us. They include Dr. Mary D. Ainsworth (professor of psychology at The Johns Hopkins University), Mrs. Franc Balzar (former national director of Parent-Child Centers of the U.S. Office of Child Development), Dr. Frank Falkner (professor of pediatrics at the University of Cincinnati College of Medicine, and director of the Fels Research Institute), Dr. Jacob L. Gewirtz (chief of the Section on Early

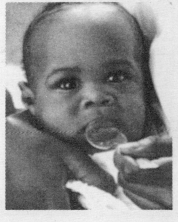

Learning of the National Institute of Mental Health in Bethesda, Maryland), the late Dr. Eric H. Lenneberg, linguist (former professor of psychology and neurobiology at Cornell University in Ithaca, New York), Dr. Michael Lewis (formerly the director of the Infant Laboratory at the Educational Testing Service in Princeton, New Jersey), Dr. Lewis P. Lipsitt (research psychologist and director of The Child Study Center at Brown University, Providence, Rhode Island), Dr. Myrtle McGraw (retired professor and director of The Baby Teaching Laboratory in closed Briarcliff College, Briarcliff Manor, New York), Dr. Frank A. Pedersen (research psychologist at The National Institute of Child Health and Human Development, Bethesda, Maryland), and Dr. Roger A. Webb (assistant professor of psychology at The Johns Hopkins University).

We are pleased to share with you the sensitive photographs taken by Ullie Steltzer, as well as the loan of delightful pictures from her personal collection of parents and babies in other countries.

Frank Caplan's deep interest in the first three years of life began in 1931, when he was probably the first male nursery school teacher in the United States at The City and Country School in New York City. I am continuing to be involved in his vision of a better life for parents and their children as the director of The Princeton Center for Infancy and Early Childhood.

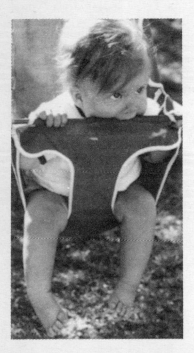

Heartfelt kudos go to Mrs. Dorothy J. Naylor for her encouragement and steadfast typing and retyping of our manuscript. We enjoyed working with Eileen Cope, assistant editor at Putnam, whose enthusiasm and interest made our efforts worthwhile. Many thanks, too, to Laura Yorke, senior editor, for her final editorial review.

We hope the years ahead will be exciting ones for new parents. Through the use of electronic devices and advanced techniques, researchers are now better able to delve into the maturation and thinking processes of infants.

THERESA CAPLAN

Contents

The Twelfth Month 357

STEPPING OUT

The joy of walking; balance; new freedom; interference
with eating and sleeping; fear of strangers; beginning of
speech; independence-dependence

Introduction

The birth of your baby begins a fascinating year of adventure for both of you, a year in which your infant learns basic rules of physical control, thought, socializing, and communicating. A baby is extraordinarily dependent on his parents in comparison to most infant animals. The imbalance between a baby's senses of sight, hearing, smell, taste, and touch and his virtual physical inadequacy often frustrate baby and parents. Luckily, he is given enough time to learn the complicated essentials of being human while he is still protected.

Infancy is a spectacular time in life. In the next twelve months, you will see your baby changing faster and working harder than at any other period in his life. He has a great deal to learn. In about half that time the little being you see now will probably begin to sit alone, reach for and grasp a toy, recognize a familiar face, smile, laugh, and hold up his end of a conversation with you by cooing and babbling. By the year's end, he will stand, probably walk, handle a toy or a spoon, say a few words, and, being a sociable person, distinguish the people in his life from the strangers, and form strong attachments to some of them. He even will have settled down to a routine of three meals a day, an afternoon nap, and sleeping through the night. He will have learned that something heard is something to see, that things seen may be grasped, and that things have permanence even when they are out of hand and sight. He will have begun to understand what part of the world is "him" and what part is not, and how to influence both parts.

How is all this accomplished? To some extent, it is a natural process of unfolding with the same sequences of stages occurring in all babies the world over. Development follows a head-down-to-toes direction. Eye muscles come under control first, then the facial muscles, neck muscles, and finally the trunk and the legs. Development also follows a center-outward-to-fingertips direction. At one stage your baby will wave his arms, use them to help him sit, and reach for toys hung over his crib. At a later stage, he will control his wrist, fingers, and thumb so that he can pick up and release things precisely.

There are variations, however, in the time at which these stages occur. Not all babies smile, sit, or reach out at exactly the same age. Do not expect your baby to conform to any rigid schedule of development. Be aware that every baby develops at his own rate, in his own style, and each is an individual.

A baby is born into the world with basic needs and drives. He wants to survive and he wants to fit into his environment. Even very young infants actively seek stimulation. Far from being passive, babies strive to master their environment and to identify with it. What happens to these drives is a product of the exchanges between every baby's unique heredity and his world.

From the moment of birth, individual differences are apparent that determine the reactions of parents to their offspring. Babies can be individual enough to want to practice their budding skills alone sometimes. Not only do they not need mother or father around, on occasion they actually do not want them. On the other hand, your baby may seem to want constant cuddling. In the early weeks, differences are less obvious than the similarity of every baby's needs, and of his responses when needs are or are not met.

The mother and father are the most critical influence in their infant's first year of life. In fact, they are their baby's primary teachers. They nurture their baby to the best of their ability, in a loving atmosphere, so that he has a good head start. They appreciate that coping with the uncertainties of later life requires suitable preparation. Children learn positive ethical and social values from their parents.

It is for these reasons and many others that this book is addressed to mothers and fathers. Both should choose the obstetrician, clinic, or health-care system for the prenatal period of their fetus. The father needs to make certain that he will be able to attend the birth, even if it is suddenly a cesarean one. He can play the major role in the support of his wife before, during, and after the birth of their baby.

The prepared childbirth movement, Lamaze for one, has furthered the active, educated involvement of the father. The obstetrician, midwife, or maternity nursing staff are encouraging the overwhelmed new father to look at, touch, and hold his wonderful baby. He learns the techniques of diapering and bottle-feeding before his wife and baby are ready to leave the hospital or the birthing center.

The quality of parenting and the interactions between parents and baby in the earliest weeks substantially determine how far development in the first year will progress. Clearly, a child whose environment allows him to develop to his fullest intellectual potential, and provides a happy, stimulating, and healthy childhood in which the capacity to love and to be loved is rewardingly learned through his earliest interactions with his parents will fare the best.

There are no strict rules to parenting. Your individual reactions, common sense, and intuition may be as right as the idealized suggestions of an "authority" may be wrong. Our parents used to be told not to pick up an infant or cuddle him; too much attention and handling would "spoil" him. Today we realize that when parents enjoy playing with their baby, it not only gives the baby pleasure, it sets a precedent for his deriving satisfaction from his relationships with other people. Each baby becomes a special experience for all parents. Young parents do better to chart their own behavior from the cues set out for them by their baby. The broad outlines of growth and development are universal, but the details have to be inscribed for each baby by parents who are sensitively responsive to his particular needs at each stage of his life.

Once parents recognize the wide range of normal infant behavior, they will better understand the how and why of each step in development that this book describes. It helps to know that their baby's state—whether he is crying, drowsy, active, or alert—influences his responses during the hectic first three months far more than it does later on; also, that a baby cries not because he is angry at mother or father; rather, he is frustrated by his inability to grapple

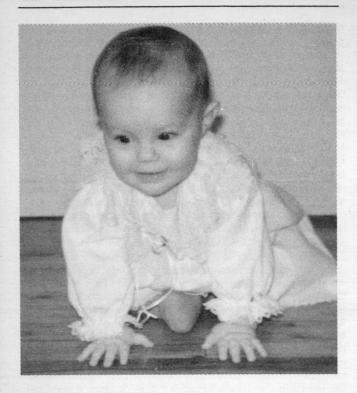

with elements in a world he is gradually becoming aware of. Parents in the United States need to know more about child care. Without the guidance and support of the grandparents, aunts, uncles, and cousins of yesteryear's extended family, they are alone with their baby for long stretches of time.

Besides stressing the role and value of parent-child interactions, and the importance and influence of the environment, each chapter in this book features a special event most likely to appear in that or a neighboring month, even though the topic may be touched on elsewhere. We have not portrayed an "average" mean because the averages were computed decades ago and, again, because we have tried also to acquaint you with the vast individual differences among normal babies. Because the human infant is so changeable and "unknown," we have gleaned information from books, articles, monographs, research reports, and professional papers. Infancy research is exciting, informative, and challenging. However, its research tools continue to be tentative. The strict model of laboratory settings based on structured, inflexible test situations oftentimes blurs the child's vital individuality. Therefore, we have chosen to mellow this book with the seasoned, long-term observations of outstanding scientists and pediatricians.

We cannot repeat too often that this book describes a sequence, not a timetable. Within that general framework, you and your baby will have to discover what "works" for him.

Whether you are new parents or "old hands," we would like to give you a feeling for both your infant and his world that will help you experience and enjoy him together. At the same time, we hope we can help you feel less hesitant and more sure of yourselves as mothers and fathers than our parents' generation. Parents who give of themselves and respect their children as individuals can say no as well as yes, and can confidently let go of them at the right time. In the meantime, we want to assist you in choosing a personal style of learning and living with your baby by offering you the wide spectrum of normal and expected infant behaviors and infant-rearing practices.

Raising children entails joys, frustrations, hard work, and assorted problems of minor or major proportions. Although it is not necessary to be a "perfect" parent, to be a "good enough" parent requires knowledge, patience, and experience. Parents benefit from understanding the ages and stages of the physical, emotional, and mental growth all children go through on their innate timetables. Growth cannot be pushed. The sequence of the stages of human development is more or less constant; it is the timing that is purely personal. The great spurts in coordination and learning that occur during the first twelve months of life are not replicated in the same degree and intensity in later years.

We hope that this revised and updated edition of *The First Twelve Months of Life* will help you both enjoy this challenging time together.

Before the First Week

GENERAL INFORMATION FOR
MOTHERS AND FATHERS

Before your baby is born, you might want to know certain information to make you feel comfortable about what you will encounter in your child's first few hours, days, and months. This chapter offers overall information to give you some quick, reassuring knowledge if you are a first-time parent.

Cesarean Birth

When preparing for the birth of their babies, most women and men think only in terms of vaginal birth. Sometimes, however, the obstetrician is faced with the need to do a cesarean section. Included among the various reasons for this procedure are: the premature separation of the placenta from the woman's uterine wall; the baby's head is too large to pass through the birth canal; the baby is lying crosswise in the mother's abdomen; the placenta is implanted on the lower part of her uterus, thus blocking the baby's exit; the umbilical cord comes through the pelvic outlet first, impeding the flow of blood and oxygen to the baby; a fibroid tumor is blocking the pelvic outlet, preventing the baby from passing through; a prolonged or difficult labor (called dystocia); the expectant mother has diabetes mellitus or a ruptured uterus.

Two types of skin incisions are used: transverse (bikini) or vertical (midline). The bikini incision has cosmetic advantages and offers greater comfort than the midline incision

1

because the abdominal muscles are less affected. Uterine incisions are done independently of the skin incision and may be transverse (in the lower segment of the uterus) or classical (vertical). The transverse is considered safest for the mother and is necessary if she is interested in delivering vaginally in a subsequent pregnancy.

The mother may have general anesthesia (which makes her unconscious during the delivery) or spinal or epidermal anesthesia (which produces a complete loss of feeling from the abdomen down). The postoperative care of the mother is similar to that of any patient who has undergone major surgery.

While being used too frequently according to many medical and childbirth experts, cesarean births may be the best option available when the baby or the mother is at risk or when complications arise.

Many obstetricians automatically deliver all breech babies via cesarean section because of the risks involved in the vaginal delivery of babies when their buttocks or feet instead of their heads appear first at the uterine outlet. Improved anesthesia, surgical techniques, and infection prevention have led to greatly reduced infant and maternal mortality rates.

Of course, there is an increased physical burden on the mother as well as emotional upset to both parents when a cesarean birth is required. However, the presence of the father in the operating room and closer contact between mother and newborn appear to assuage the new family's post-cesarean reactions. Nowadays cesarean-birth education is being added to the regular curriculum of planned childbirth classes; those of Lamaze, for one.

The norm used to be "once a cesarean, always a cesarean," but now giving birth vaginally after a cesarean is the rule rather than the exception in most cases.

Birthmarks

Various unusual marks (skin blemishes) may be present at birth or during the earliest months of life. Most are reddish, reddish-blue, or deep pink splotches across the back of the baby's neck, on the forehead, bridge of the nose, or eyelids. Some appear on various parts of the body. Caused by the slight enlargement of the infant's tiny blood vessels, most do not require treatment. Birthmarks worry parents, particularly when they are on the baby's face. Talk to your pediatrician if you are concerned. Below are descriptions of various kinds of birthmarks:

Salmon Patches or Stork Bites are deep pink splotches that usually are on the bridge of the nose, lower forehead, upper eyelids, back of the head, or neck. This most common birthmark disappears in the baby's first few months of life.

Mongolian Spots are large, flat areas that contain extra pigment. They appear on the lower back or buttocks. Very common, especially in dark-skinned babies, they usually disappear by school age.

Moles (or Nevi) are present at birth or are acquired. Composed of nevus cells, similar to those that give dark pigment to the skin, these spots are dark brown or black. Small moles present at birth are relatively common. They tend to grow with the child and usually do not cause any problems. However, it is wise to have them checked by your pediatrician at regular intervals, especially if there is any change in color, size, or shape.

Hemangiomas occur when a certain area of the skin develops an abnormal blood supply during early childhood, which in turn cause the tissue to enlarge and become reddish-blue. There are different kinds of hemangiomas.

Strawberry Hemangiomas are found in two of every hundred newborn babies. Although they often are not noticeable at birth, they can appear within the first month of life as raised red dots on any part of the body. Most commonly they are evident on the head, neck, and trunk.

If your infant develops a strawberry hemangioma, have your pediatrician examine it so he or she can follow its course. During the first six months of life, strawberry hemangiomas that grow rapidly can be quite alarming to parents. In fact, their reddish-purplish appearance so disturbs parents that they want to have them removed at once. However, most will gradually reduce in size over the second to third year of life and ultimately disappear.

Strawberry hemangiomas may need to be treated or removed when they occur close to the eye, throat, or mouth, or when they seem to be growing very fast. Have your doctor evaluate the condition every time he or she checks your baby.

Port Wine Stains (or flat hemangiomas) usually are present at birth and enlarge as the child grows. Dark red, they are found on the face or limbs, usually on one side of the body. These hemangiomas do not go away, although they sometimes fade, and they rarely cause any problems. Port wine stains should be examined by your doctor from time to time to evaluate their size, location, and appearance.

An Infant's Basic Senses

The following information is presented to give you a general overview of what you can expect, and to offer a few reasons why early sensory stimulation is so important.

HEARING

Not only do newborns hear at birth, they are now assumed to hear while in utero. Many pregnant women report that their unborn babies jerk suddenly at a loud noise. Often mothers attending a concert can feel the fetus moving more than usual. Thus, it may never be too soon to expose your baby to music and pleasant sounds. Avoid loud rock music or too many people in your infant's room because they will shut out his ability to distinguish one sound from another. Distinguishing sounds (attending and associating) is an important learning process. If the room is constantly full of sounds that cannot be differentiated, the infant gives up listening and differentiating.

There has been considerable research on the hearing ability of newborns. Neonates from twenty-seven to seventy-seven hours old definitely react to sound stimuli. If your baby does not respond to a loud sound, it does not necessarily indicate a hearing impairment. Many babies are born with fluid in their ears that produces temporary "deafness." This condition usually clears up in a short time.

At two months of age, a baby can recognize his mother's

voice. If he is fussing and upset, others may try comforting him, but nothing seems to be as effective as his mother's voice and handling. This also is the age when a baby starts to locate sounds. Inasmuch as hearing is one of the most important senses used in acquiring information, it is important that you stimulate your baby very early.

Several ways to provide this stimulation might be to:

1. Hang a small, brightly colored plaything with a securely attached bell in the crib. Make sure it is near enough (seven inches from his eyes) so the three-month-old baby can strike it when he waves his hands. This will not only exercise his listening, but will also afford him an opportunity to observe a simple cause/effect relationship. The baby discovers that the movement of his arm or other body parts can elicit sound from the object.

2. Turn on a radio or phonograph softly in your baby's room. Do this several times a day. This may be a good way to end your baby's day also. When you turn out his light at night, turn on a music box.

3. Sing to your baby.

4. Hold your baby close to a piano while someone plays softly.

5. Talk, talk, talk to your baby!

SMELLING

The sense of smell is often overlooked by both researchers and parents as another important sensory channel through which the baby may be stimulated. A baby is born with strong facial muscles and an intact smelling apparatus that are basic for survival since they are used for eating and breathing. Some of the earliest signs of learning are revealed through these sensory modalities. They are associated with stimulation of the mouth and food intake.

It is a widely held misconception that newborns cannot smell. One researcher, Dr. Lewis P. Lipsitt, has accurately studied the responses of newborn infants to smells. He and Clement A. DeLucia devised a little rubber cot stretched on steel rods and sensitized to a baby's overall body activity and bounces. They presented newborns with various substances that give off odors, and discovered that babies less than three days old can differentiate smells.

It was also noted that after repeated exposure to particular odors, babies responded less and less to subsequent presentations of those odors.

SEEING

Although much remains unknown about the visual world of the newborn, we have come a long way in a relatively short time span. It was not so long ago that journals were advising parents not to be concerned about their baby's vision because he could not "see" until about six months of age. The fact is that certain basic visual powers function in the newborn, powers that become important tools for communication and learning.

Absent at birth is the ability of the baby's head and eyes to work in unison; the head will lag behind as the eyes follow a moving object. However, the newborn can fixate briefly on stable objects and tentatively follow a slow-moving object with both eyes through fairly short arcs.

Newborns react to light intensity, patterns, and color. They stare intently at a human face several inches away. During the earliest months of life, although they are greatly uncoordinated, babies are receptive to sensory stimulation and observe their surroundings for most of their waking hours.

Newborns react to a bright light shining in their eyes by tightly shutting their lids. They appear to prefer objects of intermediate brightness and medium complexity to objects that are too bright and very complex in design. Generally, newborns can accommodate visually at a distance of about seven inches. After several weeks, more flexible focal distances are in evidence. In the fourth month, their visual accommodation is more nearly that of the adult.

Eye examinations are recommended at birth for the inspection of birth defects (if any); at six months for the diagnosis of any persistent or marked deviation of one eye; at one year for diagnosis of coordinated movements of both eyes without deviation of one eye; and at any time if problems are observed. Screening tests for visual acuity detect not only poorly focused images, but also poor function caused by any abnormality or disease.

The research of Dr. Robert L. Fantz of Western Reserve University reveals that from birth human infants do discriminate and have certain preferences; i.e., visual patterning is more stimulating to them than color and brightness. By the age of three months, complex and novel patterns are preferred. Infants look significantly longer at a checkerboard or bull's-eye pattern than at a black square, circle, or triangle. Infants from four days to six months old look longest at a real face, somewhat less at a scrambled face, and typically ignore a black patch.

Physical Growth

Each month your baby gains approximately one to two pounds and grows half an inch. Thus, he usually will double his birth weight by five months of age. By the time your baby has reached twelve months, if he has been nourished properly, he will probably have tripled his birth weight and grown approximately ten inches.

Sleep Habits

Most newborns sleep about sixteen hours a day, divided into three- or four-hour naps spaced evenly between their feedings. Each period includes relatively equal amounts of REM (rapid eye movement) and non-REM sleep. Active dreaming occurs during REM sleep. Non-REM sleep covers four phases: drowsiness, light sleep, deep sleep, and very deep sleep, at which time the baby is almost motionless. As the infant grows older, he has non-REM sleep before entering REM sleep. The latter pattern lasts throughout adulthood.

By four months, your baby should sleep through at least one nighttime feeding; perhaps through the entire night. He should be able to go at least eight hours without being fed. If your baby is still sleeping in your room, by six months it's time to move him out. He may be awakening because he hears you or senses your presence when you are nearby.

At this stage, he needs to be in a full-size crib with protective bumpers. A night-light may add to your baby's comfort.

At eight months, your baby may continue to take a nap in the morning and one in the afternoon. He may sleep as much as twelve hours at night without requiring a middle-of-the-night feeding. Do not use a pacifier. If he needs it to fall asleep, he will cry for you each time it falls out of his mouth.

It is not a good idea to take your baby into your bed to sleep because such a pattern is not easily broken and can become a nuisance.

Feeding Overview

Dr. Myron Winick, in his introduction to Chapter 3, "Feeding and Nutrition," in *The Parenting Advisor*, states that: "It is becoming more and more evident that nutrition at critical times during the life cycle will not only stamp its mark on the organism, but also may leave a permanent legacy in time to come. Certainly infancy and early childhood are extremely critical times in this regard."

Dr. Winick, who has written countless scientific articles on nutrition, is an authority in the field. He maintains that children who have been severely undernourished in their early infancy may have learning disabilities later on in their lives because "the number of brain cells may be reduced, the insulation around the nerve fibers may be thinner than normal, the number of connections between nerves may be fewer, and the chemical milieu in which nerve impulses are delivered may be disturbed."

Overfeeding, on the other hand, may result in the creation of an overabundance of fat cells, which can result in the kind of obesity that is very hard to control.

With the advice of your pediatrician, your infant's instincts, and your own good judgment, you can forward the proper growth and development of your offspring. For instance, the healthy breast-fed baby will determine how much milk to take to grow properly. While babies can be fed adequately by breast or bottle, parents need to avoid the tendency to make sure every bottle of formula is completely consumed; more fat babies are bottle-fed than breast-fed.

The Importance of Record Keeping

The ideal time to start a family health record is before you begin your family. Record all the data you can secure about yourselves (wife and husband), your parents, siblings, grandparents, aunts, uncles, et cetera. Be sure to include in your family tree the date and place of birth, medical history, and cause of death of your close kin. The most accurate family medical history can be the key that will provide diagnosis without hours of time-consuming and costly detective work.

When you are to become parents, record all the details of the pregnancy, and then the complete natal history of your baby. There are improved baby record-keeping books on the market today, or you can create your own with a sturdy loose-leaf book or a Manila file folder.

It is a good idea to have a copy of your child's birth certificate, which can be done by photostating the original. A certified copy can be obtained from the vital statistics department of the city in which your baby was born. The original birth certificate should be kept in a fireproof place (such as a safe deposit box). Not only will you need to present it upon your child's admission to grade school, but it will also be needed by your adult offspring for obtaining a passport and other documents.

You might wish to obtain the Apgar Score of your newborn from your physician. Remember to note your baby's blood type.

It is of prime importance to keep precise data on your baby's immunizations. However, for the parent who slips up occasionally, missing information can be obtained from the pediatrician. Periodic medical findings should always be noted, because it is as helpful to know when your child has been well as when he has been ill.

Allergies and other physical problems that require special medication should be noted, along with the name of your pharmacy. (Federal law requires all pharmacies to keep up-to-date records on family prescription needs.) The information can be crucial in an emergency, and may also be helpful in a routine consultation (i.e., allergies to antibiotics, et cetera).

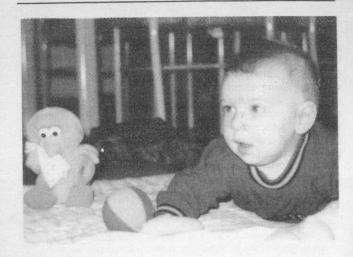

No record would be complete without regular notations on your baby's height and weight. These readings are not uniform; rather, they indicate special spurts of growth during the first year of life. (Often a doctor will check a sick child's weight before prescribing medication because dosage level is based on a child's weight.)

It is not only fun but also important to note when your baby took his first steps or said his first words. These are all factors in his development and indicate how good his motor control is.

Any injuries should be recorded at the time they happen, as well as any remarks of the attending physician, treatment, and your child's recovery.

Mementos of happy events are a special part of your child's and your life. Therefore, you will want to include in your file snapshots and perhaps a lock of hair from your child's first haircut.

What better gift could you give your infant-grown-to-adult offspring than his or her very own personal history of childhood growth and development? Everyone delights in childhood and family reminiscing and happy memories.

* * *

A word about gender. Writers on child care may someday succeed in introducing into the language a word that means both "he" and "she." Meanwhile, we will use the convention of the masculine pronoun. However, be assured that unless we are talking about something where one's sex makes a difference, everything we write about "him" refers to your new daughter as well. Similarly, until the English language invents a better term for brother and sister, you will occasionally find the word "sib," a borrowing from social science literature that means either.

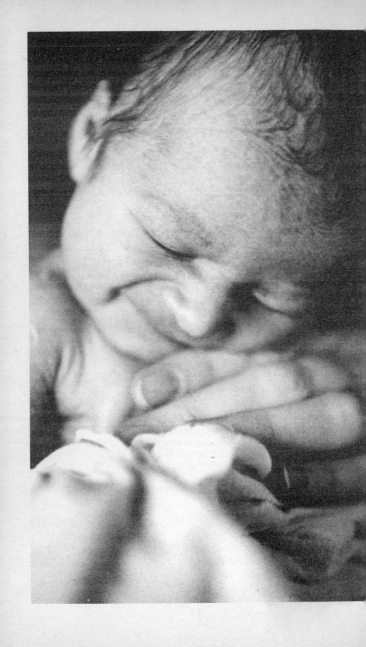

The First Week

THE NEWBORN

The Beginning Family

At birth, a baby brings much joy, work, disruption, and worry. Often parents are not ready emotionally or physically for the impact of their demanding, albeit exhilarating addition. Even though they have prepared for the baby by buying clothes, choosing a crib, discussing names, making arrangements for help, and going faithfully for prenatal checkups and to parenting education classes, most parents are jolted when they are alone at home with their infant for the first time. This feeling of unease is normal, especially for first-time parents.

Parents love their children and are eager to be "good" parents. Wanting to do what is best, they read books and articles on feeding, sleeping, child care, and much more. Nonetheless, they can become tired, nervous, and irritable. When this occurs, communication and understanding often break down between a husband and wife and the situation can get out of hand.

All new parents react deeply to the dramatic change in their lives that comes with the addition of a new family member. Many complex physiological and psychological changes affect new mothers, but complicated changes also occur in fathers when their babies are born. Psychologically the birth of a first child marks a sharp turning point in the life of every man and woman. After mother and baby come home from the hospital, many mothers experience a loss of their personal freedom. They are temporarily stunned by the realization that they can no longer do what they want when they feel like doing it. They soon learn that a visit to the theater now involves more than a phone call to reserve tickets. They cannot make plans for themselves only; now the baby's needs must also be considered.

In *Pregnancy, Birth and the Newborn Baby*, Shirley Stendig Ehrlich writes: "Enriching and gratifying as parenthood is, it also takes a toll on the previous intimacy between husband and wife. No longer is there the exclusively one-to-one relationship between husband and wife, with all the possibilities of unlimited energy for intimacy, companionship and shared activities." All new mothers and fathers would benefit from taking a three-dimensional view of their changed way of life. Beginning parents need to learn to understand and cope with the conflicting feelings and attitudes with which they are abruptly beset.

Although spouses may have worked out a sharing of household tasks and responsibilities while both were working prior to becoming parents, the new role of being parents may alter such an understanding. The husband may expect his wife to assume more (or all) of the household duties if she is at home with the baby. Also, although husband and wife may have talked about sharing the care of the baby, the husband's beginning unease at handling an infant, coupled with the wife's subconscious attitude that child care is a mother's role, may lead to ambivalence. Open communication between the parents and flexibility in both appear to be two of the most salient elements for establishing an equitable sharing of responsibilities.

Traditionally, the mother has been the primary nurturing figure, but studies indicate that the father-child interaction positively affects a child's present and future behavior. In fact, a close relationship with father during the first several years of life is critically important to the child's formation of a rounded personality and a healthy sexual identity.

Furthermore, many mothers find that they are better able emotionally to meet the needs of their babies when they derive satisfaction from pursuing their own interests. Increasing numbers of women are fulfilling themselves in activities that take them out of the home: employment, volunteerism, recreation. As a baby grows more mature physically and emotionally, and in such areas as self-help, verbal communication, and the ability to delay gratification, a patient caregiver like Dad may be able to take over.

The Nuclear Family

Each marriage marks the start of a new conjugal or nuclear family. Today's American family is a blend of traditional forms introduced to this country by various migrating cultures. The family has been modified by changes brought about by industrialization, as well as today's new sexual/social values. Family forms have changed to fit the needs of men and women in a changing society.

In his book *Are Parents Bad for Children?* Dr. Graham B. Blaine, Jr., expresses his belief that increased sexual permissiveness and the women's liberation movement

Fathers' Rights and Obligations

1. Fathers are involved, too. By attending prenatal courses with their wives, fathers are learning about adjusting to their pregnant wives' moods, the miracle of birth, and the practicalities of caring for a newborn.

2. Fathers have feelings, too. Most new mothers turn to their husbands for extra emotional support at this time, and most husbands are able and happy to provide the needed understanding and help. At the same time, many new mothers tend to isolate their husbands, and give them a minimum of attention and care. Sometimes even the most loving husbands may experience anxiety, frustration, and resentment.

3. Fathers are competent, too. They should be involved in baby care right from the start. Awkwardness and feelings of inadequacy lessen with practice, which translates into comfortable, mutually enjoyable bathing, feeding, strolling, and playing with baby.

threaten the traditional family. Today many women want to leave their homes and fulfill themselves in professional or other pursuits. He fears that if women do not feel the need for children because they prefer careers, an important segment of our population will not be perpetuated. Dr. Blaine suggests that it might be better for child-rearing chores to be undertaken by trained caregivers, because such arrangements might provide better care for children and more freedom for both parents to develop their skills.

Having the greatest impact on the family, however, are those changes that occur within the family itself. The extended family is practically extinct, leaving in its place the nuclear family consisting of a mother, father, and a child or children. Families are more democratic, with the wife and husband having equal control of family matters.

The family is a child's first social group. Each child has to learn to relate to different people with their individual personalities, insecurities, and needs. These relationships are not easy for a child to master. A consistent caregiver must act as a mediator to encourage a child to function optimally. Parents cannot take this responsibility lightly.

We are seeing varied family arrangements: nuclear families, unmarried couples, single-parent units, as well as men and women who, while they may choose to live outside the traditional family, are creating new variations on the old family theme. Each alternative appears to fill a need in the people who are drawn to it. Perhaps we need to take up the challenge of sociologists to rethink the institution of the family and to work within it rather than to discard it.

Single-Parent Family

The single-parent family is one of today's realities that appears to be here to stay. It is less a cause than a result of such social problems as economic disadvantage, racial discrimination, limited education, unemployment, and more. The high divorce rate and teenage pregnancies have exacerbated the prevalence of the one-parent household. For the most part, single parents face an uphill battle to combine making a decent living with raising children. It is difficult to be a parent in any kind of family, but child-rearing is

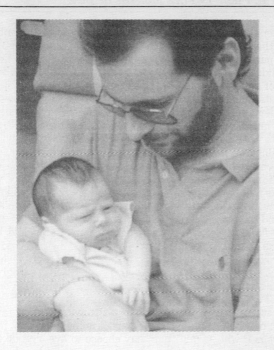

especially arduous for the single parent. Feelings of exhaustion, isolation, and frustration abound, not to mention the extreme monetary difficulty many single mothers face.

About one in five children in the United States spends at least a portion of childhood in a single-parent family. With only one parent on hand, there is added strain when that parent must work. There is sufficient data to indicate that babies and young children do better in a home with two adults rather than only one.

Bringing up a child without a partner is not easy for the one parent or the child, but as a social convention it is a little less burdensome now than it has been. Once criticized for placing personal happiness above the needs of their offspring, single parents of both sexes (whether unmarried or divorced) are finding increasing social acceptance and understanding.

According to Carole Klein, author of *The Single Parent Experience*, "Some people will probably go on to reject the idea of family entirely, choosing to live in total independence. Other people will live in groups. . . . Social theorists say that if marriage is to survive at all . . . it is absurd to think we can continue to declare only one pattern of living legitimate." Some child-rearing experts believe that children may develop better in a harmonious single-parent family than in an intact family torn by tension and conflict. There will have to be more research in this area.

Single parents need a strong support network, whether from relatives, friends, neighbors, or organized groups. Of course, single parents miss the sharing of responsibility and decision making that usually come with marriage. Also, even more than other parents, single parents are always short of time. All too often single parents harbor a strong sense of guilt on the job and at home.

Stepparent Family

According to statistics, over half a million adults become stepparents every year in the United States. Through remarriage after divorce or death, and through the first marriage of previously unwed women and men, there are about one million new stepchildren in America annually. Stepfamily interaction involves all the issues found in biological families and more, since additional relationships occur in the former. Much of the success of second marriages depends upon how well the couple adjusts to the offspring of the first union, and how smoothly the children accept their new family constellation; no mean feat for all involved.

A family that has suffered the loss of one parent (due to death, desertion, separation, divorce, or long-term hospitalization) experiences a period of transition during which the children and the remaining parent undergo painful, demanding readjustments to a different way of life. The remaining mother or father becomes of greater emotional importance to the children at a time when that parent can least afford the extra demands.

During this time, most young children regress in their development and behavior. Some withdraw and express only a rigid desire to please. Others exhibit various patterns of rebellion and negativism; for example, they may develop temper tantrums. This transitional period of adjustment is inevitable for all involved families. However, just how hard and long lasting it is depends upon the makeup of each family member.

The Interracial Family

Today there is much less censure of interracial couples and their offspring, although taboos persist. It is possible to have harmony between parents of disparate backgrounds, whether the differences are racial, ethnic, religious, or cultural. Maintaining family harmony while encouraging appreciation of differences can be social and emotional tightrope-walking, but comfortable balance can be achieved with patience, tolerance, and understanding. Differences can be celebrated rather than denigrated in the home and the community.

Parenting Together

There are at least two types of shared-caregiving families: those in which fathers are not employed in the work force and take care of the children while the mothers are employed outside the home, and those families in which both parents are employed, but they organize their work hours to permit them to assume shared responsibility for the care of their children. In such families, most fathers are involved in the daily care of their children (not a very common occurrence). Of course, shared child care is more feasible when both parents have flexible hours of employment, thus permitting them to organize their jobs around the needs of their family and themselves.

Most parents are able to promote a secure relationship with a healthy, agreeable baby, but only very patient and sensitive parents can relate to a tense, difficult baby. Researchers have found that parents who have cranky infants are more likely to experience less satisfaction in their marital lives than couples who are rearing contented, thriving babies. For the optimal development of their children, moth-

The "Good-Enough Parent"

In his book *The Natural Way to Raise a Healthy Child*, psychoanalyst Hiag Akmakjian describes what is needed to be a "good enough parent," a phrase first used by pediatrician-psychologist Dr. O. W. Winnicott to describe parents who do things fairly well, who are nonetheless far from perfect. Good-enough parents do not panic easily; they are neither intrusive nor aloof. Dr. Akmakjian maintains that "good-enough parents are attuned to baby's needs and feel empathy." They sense that normal development results in large measure from letting nature take its course. Above all, they do not smother their babies. They allow them sufficient space, time, and suitable privacy even when very young.

ers and fathers together need to be "good enough parents" first and gender representatives second.

The Newborn

A mother-in-waiting often imagines her first baby to be like the delightful three- or four-month-olds she has been admiring in magazines. She soon discovers at birth or the first feeding that nothing could be further from the truth. But balancing this rude awakening is a marvelous discovery— her baby is neither the helpless nor the unindividualized human neophyte he was once "scientifically" described to be.

Delivery is as difficult for the baby as it is for the mother. It is a battle lasting anywhere from four to twenty-four hours, from which the new arrival emerges splattered with his mother's blood and a thick, greasy, white material called vernix, which lets him slip through the birth canal.

He is no beauty. His skin may be discolored. The skin itself is wrinkled and loose and often ready to scale in creased places, such as hands and feet. Some newborns have extra stores of flesh, part of which is fluid, that make them look fat. This condition helps to tide the infant over until he can eat. As the extra padding disappears during the first week, it leaves the skin peeled and cracked, as the photograph on page 28 shows.

Besides the hair on his head, dark, fine hair called "lanugo" may cover the newborn's body. This hair matted with vernix gives him a strange pasted look. Even his cheeks, ears, shoulders, and back may be furry. Lanugo, a leftover from our monkey ancestors, disappears at the latest about the fourth month of life, leaving the baby soft and smooth.

The newborn's head is also not the most attractive in the world. It may be swollen at the top because of pressure against the pelvic outlet during the last hours of labor, and it is often molded like a melon with a point at the back. However, since mother's pelvis is usually an inch narrower than the circumference of her baby's head, this molding is quite useful. It allows the skull bones to overlap, with no damage to the brain, so the fetus's head can emerge from the mother successfully.

Generally the newborn's physical description reads like a prizefighter's. His face may be puffy and bluish; his ears may be pressed to his head in bizarre positions—for example, matted forward on his cheeks; his nose, flattened and skewed to one side by the squeeze through the pelvis; his eyes puffy; his eyelids swollen; and his temples and cheeks temporarily bruised if the obstetrician used forceps.

Bowlegs from his position in the womb are usual, and his feet may look "wind-blown" or be cocked pigeon-toed from being up beside his head for so long. They can be flexed and put in a normal position at birth.

As if this struggle were not enough, the battered arrival must, for his very life, be manhandled further. The obstetrician cuts the umbilical cord, which is the most predominant part of the newborn's abdomen. The cord stump gradually shrivels, dries, and falls off, usually from ten to twenty days after birth. The umbilical cord must be kept dry and not covered by diapers. The obstetrician then sucks the newborn's airways with a bulb-section. From then on, the baby's head is kept down. Even though it appears unnecessary for babies who cry and breathe readily upon delivery, this suction is vital. Otherwise the first breath may draw fluid and mucus farther into the lungs, making the baby gag, his breathing slow, and his temperature drop. The

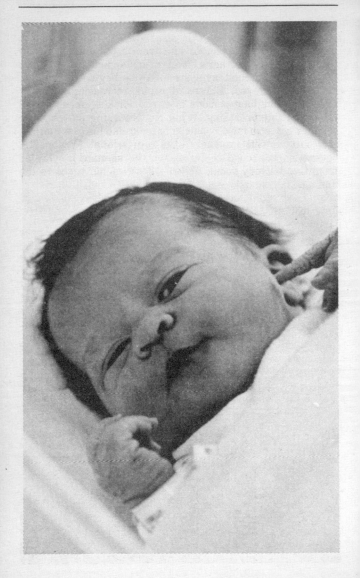

baby's first gasping cry, which the obstetrician may encourage with the classic slap, is also vital. It fills the baby's lungs with air and changes him from a parasite living off the oxygen in his mother's blood to an independent organism with his own circulatory system. As he begins to breathe, his color improves. Bursts of rapid, increasingly deeper breaths follow long periods of gasps, chokes, sneezes, and no perceptible breathing. While his breathing patterns are frightening to an inexperienced listener like his new mother, they are perfectly normal to the professional. Wrapped in several sheets to keep him warm, the neonate is wheeled from the delivery room, and the obstetrician turns to the mother.

THE APGAR SCORE

Your baby is evaluated at birth on the basis of the Apgar Score, which judges overall appearance and color, pulse rate, reflexes, muscle tone, and respiration. Developed by pediatrician Virginia Apgar, the table enables those attending a birth to assess the condition of a newborn sixty seconds or so after the birth on a score up to ten. A second evaluation is done five minutes later. A score of seven or

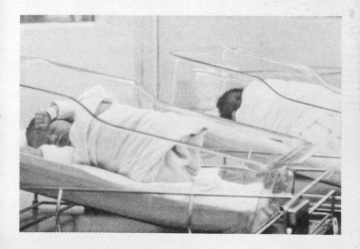

higher means your baby is in good condition. Babies who score four to six often need some oxygen administered. Those scoring below four require more extensive lifesaving measures. However, a low Apgar score even after five minutes does not necessarily signify that your baby will have neurological problems.

The First Few Days

How stunning it must be to be thrust suddenly into a new, bright, airy world so totally different from the dark, moist warmth of the womb. Despite the drama of human birth, newborns who have had a comfortable stay in the womb and are born when due can withstand even more than the usual trauma of birth. And nature allows them, unlike their mothers, a deep nourishing sleep after the contest. In the nursery, nurses rinse the blood and vernix from the infant, wash him with special medicated soap to avoid infection, and inject him with Vitamin K to prevent internal bleeding. The infant, diapered and dressed, is tilted head down in his crib. Curled in his familiar fetal position, he relaxes and falls into a deep, comalike sleep. Only the most active infants ever interrupt this. Lusty crying is very rare. Most newborns just startle, jerk briefly, or gag up mucus irregularly. Only vigorous outside stimulation disturbs them. A brief change in breathing, for example, is the only almost imperceptible response to loud noise.

In these first few days, the infant recovers from his mother's labor, the delivery, and the new stresses of the world outside the womb. Although physiologically ready to function, the infant has to stabilize his circulatory, breathing, digestion, elimination, body temperature, and hormone mechanisms, which also must start working faster for his new and independent life. Suppose *you* had been stuck in a damp sack about twenty-one inches long and a foot or so wide, in which you could hardly move and barely hear, and had no chance to breathe, smell, taste, or see anything? Then in a split second *you* have to get rid of the wastes that someone else had been relieving you of. You have to breathe for yourself in a strange world that can be cold, hot, dry, or damp. You are expected to see and to hear and can suddenly smell strange things, called odors. No wonder a baby cries when he sees his first light!

The baby's self-reorganizing leaves him little energy for eating and digesting. Many babies show this effort by actual resistance to being roused to eat. During his first days a baby is often unprepared to digest even milk, which he occasionally gags up with mucus. His stores of extra sugar, fat, tissues, and fluid sustain him until his mother's milk comes in, usually about three days or so after his delivery.

Meantime, mother herself is recovering, but she has time to think and to worry as she lies alone in her hospital bed. New mothers wonder if the baby is *really* theirs, repeatedly ask doctors and nurses for assurance that the baby is all right, worry if the baby cries too much or too little, and are often shocked by their baby's appearance. Their first response to the offspring placed in their arms is just as likely to be "My God, did I really do this?" as love at first sight.

Two of the new mother's most common concerns, pediatricians report, are about the effects of medication on the baby and the ability of the mother to nurse her infant. A woman's medication during labor, sometimes entirely necessary, does affect her infant. The effects are temporary, however. By and large, the newborn can still appear wide awake at delivery!

New mothers also wonder whether they will ever feel positively toward their new baby or whether they will be nurturing enough for him and the other children awaiting them at home. They may resent relinquishing the balance established with a first baby, doubt the new child's ability to adjust to a brother or sister, as well as their own ability to help him do this. Many feel so confused they dare not express these feelings even to themselves. Yet such conflict is natural. Giving up independence to become a mother is never easy.

Many hospital maternity staffs do little to allay a new mother's concerns. Frequently they unconsciously increase them. When a mother seeks help she is often quieted with stereotyped reassurances or condescension, even though confirmation about the normalcy of her baby can be so easy. As mentioned earlier, the Apgar test assesses whether a baby's reflexes and general physical condition are normal. A serious discussion with a doctor allows the mother to express her fears—therapeutic in itself—and permits the doctor to understand and answer her queries. Often the new mother, already coping with feelings of inadequacy, must listen to reports of others' efficiency. The inference in a nurse's classic comment—he's so quiet and good in the nursery—hardly helps a mother trying desperately to rouse her baby to nurse. Of course, one reason the baby is being difficult is that he is having a hard time, too. Remember that he is being asked to start adjusting immediately to totally new, very definite adult patterns of feeding and resting.

Yet mothering, even in the hospital, where your baby is away from you so often, can be fun. By the third day, when you and your baby have recovered a little from his dramatic entrance, you may even be able to enjoy him. Holding a little baby is lovely. Feeding periods are your chance to exercise your maternal feelings—to play, cuddle, and communicate with your baby and to begin to know him. You may find that even this early you can calm his crying or help him quiet himself with crooning or a gently placed hand. When your baby is upset, you can be an ally instead of a contestant in his struggle to feed well. Vigorous squirming may mean independence and physical sturdiness, not opposition to you. Quietness may signal resting, not disinterest.

You may even begin speculating about your infant's future coloring. Its best predictor is your own and your husband's coloring. There aren't too many other clues you can go on now. Many babies have "mongolian spots," so called because the Mongolian races usually have them, as do Negroes and brunette Caucasians. These clusters of dark pigment about the base of the baby's spine diffuse eventually and the "spots" disappear over time. Hair color is unreliable. A baby's hair falls out and is replaced by permanent hair around his fourth or fifth month. His new hair color can be dramatically different. Eye color, too, can change anytime during the first year. Almost all light-skinned babies have blue or blue-gray eyes at birth; dark-skinned infants usually have dark eyes. Six months may pass before a baby's true eye color is established.

Your newborn can see and may choose different images to look at. He can see best when things are about seven or eight inches from his eyes. He is particularly interested in the human face and bright colors. However, babies often like to keep their eyes closed.

Skin tone at birth is only a fair clue to your baby's future coloring. Most babies undergo color changes during their first week of life. From birthday purple, they gradually change to pinkish purple, to cherry red, to yellow, all of which reflect changes in the circulatory system.

Around the third day, your baby's skin and eyes may look slightly yellow or tanned, as if he had been sunning himself. Decomposing red blood cells, extras needed for the womb's lower oxygen supply in comparison to the outside air, cause this perfectly normal third-to-fifth-day jaundice. The breakdown, coupled with mild dehydration, yields a chemical called bilirubin, which the infant's immature liver just cannot get rid of. As the baby absorbs milk and his cells rehydrate, the jaundice washes out.

You will also find that your baby will eventually attain the balance he has worked so hard for. The weight he may have lost by the third day in comparison to his birthweight is all but regained, thanks to your feeding. The umbilical cord is still there but drying. He is losing his jaundiced look, his color is improving, and although the skin on his hands and feet may be cracked and peeling, he looks filled out.

Infant Power: What He Can Do with His Body

Newborns are just not as helpless as they look. First of all, the activities needed to sustain life function at birth. A newborn can breathe, suck, swallow, and get rid of wastes. He can look, hear, taste, smell, feel, turn his head, and signal for help from the first minute. Right from the start, a baby's attention can be captured by sharply contoured or circular shapes. This indicates your newborn's mental curiosity is not entirely swamped by his needs for food and comfort.

Physically, newborns are admittedly limited. A newborn is tiny. From head to heels, he may be about twenty-one inches long and weigh seven and one-half pounds. His head, about fourteen and one-half inches in circumference, is almost two thirds of his height and an inch bigger than his chest, so he is understandably awkward. Just try to imagine yourself in his shape. Even with your maturity and skill you would have a hard time getting around if your head were twice as big and your arms and legs half their size. He is bound by where you put him, and he is at the mercy of his bodily needs. His heart beats twice as fast as a grown-up's, 120 beats a minute, and he breathes twice as fast as you do, about thirty-three times a minute. He may urinate as many as eighteen times and move his bowels from four to seven times in twenty-four hours. He sleeps fourteen to eighteen hours of his twenty-four-hour day. On the average, he is alert and comfortable for only thirty minutes in a four-hour period.

Circumcision

"To circumcise or not to circumcise," that is a question that the parents of a baby boy and their doctor need to answer at birth. Routine circumcisions are performed before the baby leaves the hospital. It is customarily done as a ritual of the Jewish faith on the male baby's eighth day of life. Of course, a circumcision should be performed only on a healthy male newborn.

Circumcision is a simple surgical procedure whereby some of the foreskin that covers the tip of the penis is cut off in order to expose the tip and the opening of the urethra to air. The procedure takes only about five minutes, rarely is complicated, and does not appear to be painful beyond the initial cut. However, the wound takes several days to heal. To protect the wound, petroleum jelly or boric acid ointment on a layer of gauze is wrapped around the tip of the penis.

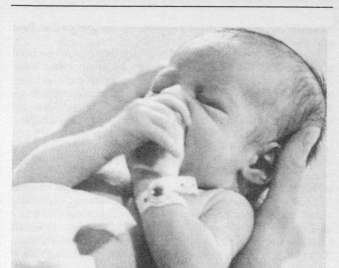

Reflexes govern his movements, which are automatic and beyond his control. For example, if you stroke your newborn's hand or foot on the back or top, the whole arm or leg withdraws slightly and the hand or foot flexes and then returns so that fingers or toes may grasp your finger. This withdrawal reflex exists only until the baby begins to use his limbs in a different way—legs for standing and stepping, arms for reaching.

There are many other reflexes your newborn will show you. If you hold him in a standing position and gently press the sole of one foot and then the other to the bed, he will draw up each leg successively as if walking. Without helping it, your newborn can actually "walk" across a bed. Almost a year after the newborn's walk reflex vanishes, it reappears as the voluntary, complex art of walking.

One of the most frequent and dramatic reflexes of the newborn is the Moro reflex, a vestige from our ape ancestry. If the baby is handled roughly, hears a very loud noise, sees a bright light, or feels a sudden change in position, he startles, arches his back, and throws his head back. At the same time, he flings out his arms and legs, then rapidly closes them to the center of his body, and flexes it as if he were falling. As he cries, he startles, then cries because of the startle. This reflex, normal in all newborns, tends to disappear at three to four months of age. Steady pressure on any part of his body will calm him. If you hold his arm firmly flexed at his shoulder, he will quiet even though undressed and free of restraints.

Try stroking different parts of your infant's body. If you stroke the palm of his hand or the sole of his foot at the base of the toes, he will grasp your finger. The more premature he is, the more tenacious his grasp. By using his toe grasp, you can lift your baby's leg off a mattress. With his hand grasp, you can gently pull him to a sitting position or even suspend him in the air hanging onto your fingers for dear life, as if to a tree branch. (Better leave this one to the experts.) Stroking the outside of the infant's sole sets off an opposite reflex, called the Babinski. The toes spread and the big toe shoots up in the air.

As you will learn as soon as you start feeding your baby, stroking his cheek or around his mouth makes him root, or turn toward the stroking object. This rooting reflex helps him find the breast, and the sucking reflex follows. Touching the inside of his mouth, which is more sensitive than the surrounding area, stimulates this reflex most. A bottle is thus easier to suck than the breast because the bottle touches this area.

Dr. Lewis P. Lipsitt of Brown University believes that babies have definite taste preferences at birth; they suck sweeter solutions faster and spit out sour ones.

If you stroke your newborn's cheek or palm—extremes of a hand-to-mouth continuum—you will start another reflex. This infant's mouth will root, his arm will flex, and his hand will come up to his open mouth. A newborn often sucks on his fist noisily for long periods (fifteen minutes or so), and so energetically that his whole body tenses and changes color until he loses his fist and random activity takes over. You need do little to start this hand-to-mouth cycle. Hand-to-mouth activity and finger sucking are probably common

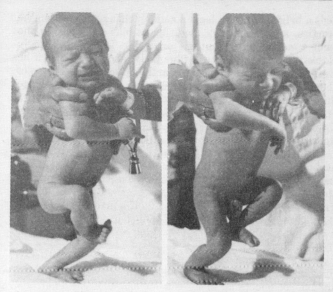

(Above) *The newborn's stepping reflex, so dramatic at birth, soon disappears and only reappears a year later as the voluntary art of walking.* (Below) *An infant has no resistance to the force of gravity. At about four months, a baby in this predicament will be able to hold his head up and try to keep his body horizontal.*

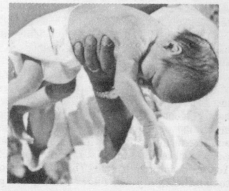

in the womb. In fact, pediatricians and obstetricians have seen these right after delivery. A premature newborn struggling to survive can actually clear his air passage by sucking on his fist and swallowing the mucus that chokes him.

Most of the newborn's remaining physical abilities are quite limited. His preferred lying-down positions vary between a rag-doll frog leg and half-extended arms to a fetal compression with all limbs pulled in. Twitches, jerky startles, and convulsive movements are the order of the day. In fact the difference between the movements of premature and full-term infants shows the importance of time and learning. The preemie's jerky flailing of limbs precedes the smooth, freely cycling, self-controlled arcs of movement of a full-term baby, who less frequently displays the preemie's movements. In contrast to slow, easy, coordinated movements of the arms, legs, and head, the baby rapidly thrusts arms and legs that suddenly flex and return to his torso.

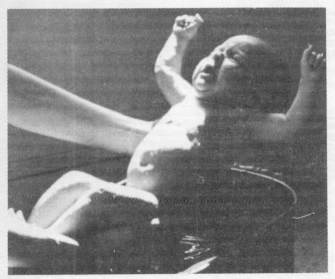

(Above) *A suddenly uncomfortable or shocking sensation triggers the Moro reflex.*

In general, the baby's responses are less specific than they will be when his nervous system is more mature. He may have the same response, such as sucking, to very different things—a light, a doorbell, or a sudden draft. He may also react with his whole body when he feels sudden changes in temperature, pressure, light, and sound.

Yet the newborn is not impotent, as the government-sponsored research of scientists like Robert L. Fantz at Western Reserve University, William Kessen of Yale, Peter Wolff of the Massachusetts Institute of Technology, and Burton White and Jerome S. Bruner of Harvard shows.

Says Dr. Fantz, "The findings to date have tended to destroy the myth that the world of the newborn is a big blooming confusion, that his visual field is a formless blur, that his mind is a blank slate. . . . The infant sees a patterned and organized world which he explores discriminatingly with the limited means at his command."

Speaking of what he called "the new look in research on infancy," Dr. L. Joseph Stone of the Department of Child Study at Vassar says, "Our conception of the newborn is changing; the neonate is more sensitive to and aware of the world, he is more responsive to it, and he is earlier influenced by his interaction with it than we had previously believed. Even his reflexes are far from the purposeless activities they were once thought to be."

The newborn can already protect himself. For several days after birth, his gag reflex helps him spit up the mucus from his mother's womb so that he can breathe. A strong blink reflex protects his eyes from too much light. If one part of his body is exposed to a sharp temperature change, his whole body changes color and temperature, he pulls in his limbs to reduce the exposed body surface, and finally begins to cry and shiver to try to improve his body's circulation and to protest this unwelcome change. As soon as he is covered and warm, he will quiet.

He can avoid smothering. If you place an object over his nose and mouth, he will mouth it vigorously and then twist his head violently from side to side. If these maneuvers fail to remove it, he will cross each arm over his face to try to knock the object off.

On his tummy, he will lift his head from the bed and turn

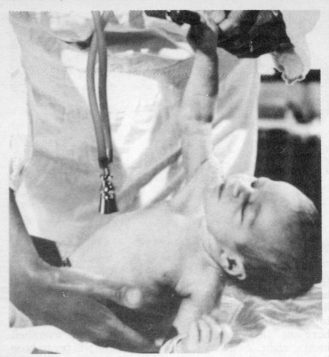

(Above) *You can gently pull a newborn to a sitting position just by drawing upon the reflexive grasp of his fingers.* (Opposite) *Another intricate reflex involving the infant's mouth, arm, and hand begins when you gently stroke his cheek.*

it to one side. Place your hand against his foot and he will crawl forward, arch his body, and even raise himself on his arms. Sometimes newborns flip themselves completely over. At this stage they are unaware of propelling themselves across space, but around the seventh month they will know what they are doing.

A newborn also tries to right himself. You will see one of your baby's righting reflexes if you pull him by his arms

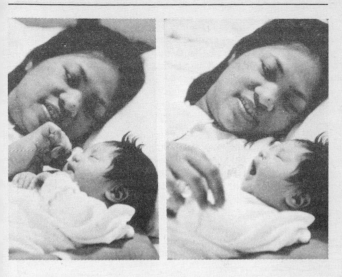

from his back to a sitting position. His eyes will open wide like a china doll's and his whole shoulder area will tense as he helps to pull up his head. As long as you pull your baby to sit slowly and steadily, the wobbling of his neck won't hurt him. Once seated, he will try to keep his oversized head upright. As his head flops forward, he will try to keep it in line, but it will "overshoot" and fall backward. As he tries again, it will tilt forward. These valiant efforts are righting reflexes. In just four months' time he will be able to hold his head upright.

The newborn can also avoid pain. If you hurt any part of him, he will withdraw from you if he can. Stroking one leg will make the other cross and push your hand away. If you poke the upper part of his body, his hand comes over to grasp yours. Then he will try to push or bat you away.

Dr. Brazelton reports that when he has to take blood from an infant's heel, "the infant will pull his foot away. When this doesn't work, the other foot comes over persistently to push."

These reflexes are not just immediately useful. Your

baby's brain stores and learns from all these reflex experiences, building for the future. The baby's righting reflexes probably contribute to the development of his concepts of space. For several months, the tonic neck reflex helps him learn to use each side of his body separately and to watch and use his hands *voluntarily*. If you or the baby turn his head to one side, the arm on the side to which his head is turned extends, the knee on that side flexes, and the opposite arm crooks like a fencer's.

Some reflexes, such as coughs, sneezes, and yawns, never go away completely, and traces of reflexes, like the tonic neck reflex and the Moro reflex, show up in adult sleep positions and in our responses to being startled. Newborns also swim reflexively. Like any amphibian, an infant can rhythmically extend and flex his arms and legs, swing his trunk from side to side, and stop breathing for short periods under water. Newborns rarely choke or breathe in water because their gag reflexes are still too strong. About a year

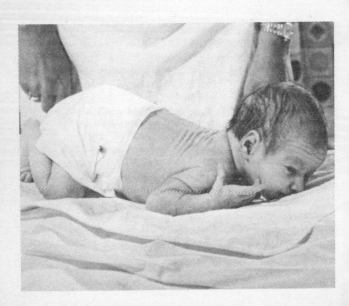

later, swimming movements will reappear and signal an opportune time to teach your toddler to swim.

Sense Perception

Even more exciting, your baby is a thinking, feeling being. True, his brain is still immature and he remembers objects only if they reappear within two and one-half seconds; otherwise they are new as far as he is concerned. So far satisfaction and displeasure are the only emotions researchers and mothers have clearly discerned. But your baby *does* learn. He learns to distinguish the nipple from the surrounding skin or bottle. He also seems able to distinguish people from objects. Researchers at Harvard's Center for Cognitive Studies write, "From the first week there seem to be features that characterize orientation to a small object . . . within six to seven inches from the eyes which are different from the features that characterize responses to people."

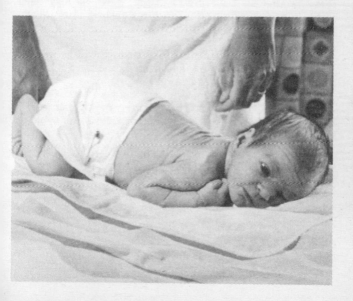

The newborn learns to expect food at a certain time and protests any change in service. Researchers' observations of three groups of infants two to eight days old showed their activity dropped sharply after nursing. Changing one group from a three-hour to a four-hour schedule made them much more active and fussy in the fourth hour than babies who had to cope with only one schedule for eight days.

Your newborn can focus his attention on a particular new thing he sees or hears—amidst a bombardment of stimulation. Doing so quiets him. He can prefer one reaction to another (at a particular moment) and can tune in or out when stimulation is appropriate or inappropriate to his particular state at that moment, or to his general stage of development. He can choose what he needs from his environment, as long as you give him something to choose from. He can suppress many potentially harmful reactions. In fact, a barrage of strong or changing events can put a newborn to sleep. An infant being given a cardiogram and brainwave test can cry with discomfort for a few seconds if rubber bands around his scalp are too tight. Then he may quiet abruptly and remain motionless throughout testing, seemingly asleep except that his arms and legs are pulled tightly into the fetal "ball." Bright lights and sharp noises barely seem to disturb him and his brainwave shows the pattern of sleep. As soon as the stimulation stops and the tight bands are off, however, he cries lustily.

The newborn's most impressive powers are sensory. Your baby can feel changes in temperature, distinguish tastes, and by the third or fourth day show preference for sweet and dislike of bitter flavors. Dr. Lewis P. Lipsitt of Brown University has shown that newborns not only can distinguish between two smells, they actually despise foul odors. In a series of experiments he discovered some amazing facts. Babies with as little as fifty-five hours of experience on earth can differentiate smells—and with no practice. When introduced to strong (irritating to adult) odors, babies become startled and very active. They will turn their heads away and cry. As they grow older, their heartbeats slow down, showing that babies get bored with the odor game or even get used to offensive odors if provided in small doses.

They are also very sensitive to touch and pressure. Touch is almost a language for infants. Skin contact and warmth, especially from mother's body, are probably the most potent stimulation for infants in the first few months of life. Like a radar screen picking up vibrations, your baby soaks in your feelings about him from your handling. He can sense rough, inappropriate, or insufficient handling, and he appreciates touch suited to his style. In fact, touch is so important that infants with caretakers who give them adequate physical stimulation and little else progress well for the first five or six months. As the late Dr. Lawrence K. Frank indicated, "One of the major reasons for defective development in institutional babies is the infrequent handling they receive." Many fussing or crying babies will quiet and become alert and interested when a hand is placed on their tummies or a foot is firmly restrained. Swaddling may be even more effective because it combines the quieting, soothing aspect of touch with firm, steady pressure.

Babies are also born hearing. Tests show that newborns blink, jerk, and draw in their breath sharply in response to sounds. They also prefer certain sounds to others. Many mothers report that music, the hum of motors, soft rhythmic drumming, and human voices calm fussy, irritable babies.

A newborn distinguishes volume. Even in the delivery room, he can startle or shudder at a loud noise, then shut it out the second or third time around. Soft noises, like crooning, produce fleeting, crooked smiles. The newborn can also localize a sound ten minutes after birth. He will become alert with a start, control his startle reaction, and turn to the sound, sometimes shifting his attention and energy completely away from an important function such as sucking. Length of a sound also affects him. He will respond to a ten-second tone but not one lasting one or two seconds. He distinguishes pitch. Research indicates that newborns, before learning can be a factor, quiet and become alert more consistently in response to a high-pitched than a low voice—possibly in readiness for mother's rather than father's voice.

One of the most exciting discoveries of the growth sciences has been that young infants are visually sophisticated organisms. Newborns see. A newborn will alert, frown, and gradually try to focus on a red or soft yellow object dangled about eight to twelve inches before him. Beyond that range, he probably has only a hazy image and his eyes may wander independently or flair outward for a while. Once he gets his eyes together, he will stare intently at the object, eyes glistening. His face will brighten and his body quiet. He will follow, or track, the object with his eyes and turn his head slowly and jerkily when the object is moved slowly from side to side. He can even follow it up and down if it moves very slowly. This visual responsiveness is evident even in the delivery room. Since his experience with vision has been zero in the womb, you know he is born seeing. In fact, some newborns delight so much in seeing, they will actually drop the nipple and turn to an attractive object.

The newborn is also sensitive to other visual matters, such as the intensity of light. He will shut his eyes tightly and keep them shut after being exposed to a bright white light. He will squint if the light in a room changes.

He can discriminate shapes and patterns (the arrangements of lines and details) from birth. He prefers patterns to dull or bright solid colors and looks longer at stripes and angles than at circular patterns. Within three weeks, however, his preference shifts dramatically to the human face. Why should a baby with so little visual experience attend more to a human face than to any other kind of pattern? Some scientists think this preference represents a built-in advantage for the human species. The object of prime importance to the physically helpless infant is a human being. Babies seem to have an inborn tendency to perceive the human face as potentially rewarding. Researchers also point out that the newborn wisely relies more on pattern than on outline, size, or color. Pattern remains stable, while outline changes with point of view; size, with distance from an object; and brightness and color, with lighting. Facial pattern is probably the most reliable way to identify people under different circumstances, and the best way to judge their reactions and attitudes is by the details of their facial expression. This "imprinting" of the human face is an important basis for all subsequent learning and for the growth of attachment and love.

Mothers have always claimed that they could see their newborns looking at them as they held them, in spite of what they have been told. The experts who thought that perception had to await physical development and the consequence of action were wrong for several reasons. Earlier research techniques were less sophisticated than they are today. Physical skills were once used to indicate perception of objects—skills like visual tracking and reaching for an object, both of which the newborn does poorly. Then, too, assumptions that the newborn's eyes and brain were too immature for anything as sophisticated as pattern recognition caused opposing data to be discarded or misinterpreted. Since perception of form was widely believed to follow perception of more "basic" qualities such as color and brightness, the possibility of its presence from birth was discounted out of hand.

How *your* baby responds to sights, sounds, and touch depends on their intensity, his length of exposure to them, and also his state at the time. Sudden jarring will cause a startle, but rhythmic rocking soothes. When hungry or sleepy, he is less aware of sensations from the outside world than in moments of quiet but alert wakefulness, when he feels no discomfort from within.

Feeding Baby

The expectant mother has to consider the relative merits of breast- and bottle-feeding so she can decide which method will be best in her case. The specific feeding practice you use—breast or bottle, schedule or demand—matters less emotionally than the context of the mother-child relationship. The only kind of feeding generally frowned on is propping the bottle, because the baby misses the warm security and pleasure of human contact. Some pediatricians feel this lack can seriously interfere with his chance for normal psychological development. Being alone with a bottle is a cold way for an infant to experience such an important daily event and forces him to rely on his own resources at feeding time. This reliance is apt to prolong and intensify his attachment to his bottle since he has had to turn to it as his primary gratification when feeding.

With that exception, the most thorough scientific attempt to date to compare the effects of breast-feeding with those of bottle-feeding concluded that factors such as the sex of the baby and the warmth or rejection of the mother were more important than the style of feeding. What seems critical is the kind and amount of sensory and social stimulation a mother gives her baby and her gratification of his needs. Bottle-feeding and breast-feeding both give the baby the security and tactile stimulation of being held and supported, as well as the social stimulation of being talked to and played with.

Even so, there are decided differences between breast- and bottle-feeding. Although bottle-feeding is preferred by the great majority of mothers, increasing numbers are returning to the natural custom that has many advantages for infant and mother alike.

THE CASE FOR BREAST-FEEDING

Breast-feeding gives the most opportunity for close contact between mother and child. The greatest asset to the mother may be a kind of peace within herself during and after nursing. Mothers say they feel they have given their babies a real part of themselves, have communicated on the baby's terms for a short time, and do not feel guilty leaving them for the next few hours to tend to other children and responsibilities. Furthermore, today most experts believe that on the basis of nutrition alone, breast milk generally is superior to any formula. Breast-feeding gives infants an available-on-demand combination of carbohydrates, protein, fat, minerals, and vitamins. At the same time, breast milk contains infection-fighting substances that help protect newborns against bacterial and yeast infections. Most doctors believe breast milk can be the main source of food for the first six months of a baby's life. To recap the benefits of breast-feeding:

1. Immediacy: breast-feeding requires no preparation.
2. Nutrition: breast milk contains the most complete nutritional package which is fresh and sterile.
3. Digestibility: breast milk, which digests easily and rap-

idly, promotes the growth of desirable bacteria in the baby's digestive system, giving excellent immunity in the first few months of life.

4. Simplicity: the baby is always in control; his sucking regulates the amount of milk he drinks.

5. Economy: there is no waste with breast-feeding.

6. Nurturing: the mother can concentrate on nursing, during which a unique psychological bond develops between her and her baby.

Also, breast-fed babies are less likely to overeat. Of course, breast-feeding is less costly than formula and, in many ways, more convenient. There is no formula to buy or make, no concerns about sterility or clean water, and no extra supplies to take along when away from home.

Breast-feeding does require the nursing mother's continuing responsibility to maintain a well-balanced diet that is high in nutrients. It is important that breast-feeding mothers reduce or eliminate alcohol and caffeine from their diets, and give up smoking, because nicotine and other chemicals accumulate in breast milk.

There are other doubts that may plague an expectant mother as she contemplates how best to feed her newborn. If she decides to try breast-feeding, she may fear that her milk supply will be insufficient in quality or amount. She may wonder how to go about nursing her baby in a public place. She may be concerned that her husband or other relatives and friends may have definite opinions as to the desirability of one method over another. It is important to discuss these issues with a knowledgeable individual. When parents meet with their obstetrician or when they visit the maternity wing of the hospital prior to delivery, they should be prepared to ask questions about a feeding regimen for their new baby.

The breast-feeding mother needs to consume 500 more calories than the amount needed to maintain her normal body weight, and to drink plenty of water daily. Breast-fed infants can become hyperactive and wakeful if their mothers consume too much caffeinated beverages, including coffee, tea, colas, hot chocolate.

One very useful source for mothers who desire information on the techniques of breast-feeding is the La Leche League International, with its national headquarters at 9616 Minneapolis Avenue, Franklin Park, IL 60131. There are local chapters in many areas. This organization provides excellent literature for parents who desire information about breast-feeding.

If after discussing the pros and cons of breast- versus bottle-feeding with your doctor, husband, and friends you are still undecided about which feeding technique is right for you, why choose at all? Many women consider the combination of breast-feeding plus an occasional bottle to be the best approach. Regardless of the technique you use, you should feel happy and secure when you are feeding your infant. It is much more important that a feeling of confidence and contentment be conveyed to your newborn than where the milk is coming from.

HOW TO BREAST-FEED

First of all, relax! You have chosen to feed your newborn in the most natural way, one that will afford both of you special intimacy. You can feel confident that your milk will be just perfect for your baby. As an added bonus, there will be no need for you to worry about allergies, digestive upsets, formula preparations, sterilization, et cetera.

During pregnancy your breasts have probably become larger and your nipples darker in preparation for breast-feeding. Your nipples, which have the largest sweat glands of all, are partially sterile. Newly secreted human milk is said to have an antibacterial action. Therefore, the nipples are ready for sucking whenever the baby needs to be fed. While general cleanliness of the mother is a given, no special cleansing before or after nursing is really necessary. In fact, too much washing can cause the nipples to become dry. Should this happen, you will need to use a special cream to keep your nipples soft.

Some doctors recommend regular, gentle massage of the nipples during the last month of pregnancy to toughen them. For a large majority of women, it is probably not necessary. Your nipples may be slightly tender during the first feeding or two, just from the suction your baby applies to receive his food. This discomfort seldom continues, particularly as you learn to relax and your milk flows readily.

During the eighth month of pregnancy, or perhaps earlier in some mothers, and in the first four to five days after delivery, there is a considerable amount of secretion from the breast which is known as *colostrum*. This colostrum is a nutritional powerhouse for your baby.

Procedure

In order to be fed efficiently, your baby needs to have more of your breast in his mouth than just the nipple. Your baby has an instinctive reaction to turn his head and open his mouth toward whatever is touching his cheek. He will become confused and annoyed if you try to forcefully move his head toward your breast. However, if you lightly stroke his cheek with your finger or your nipple, he will turn his head and with your thumb and forefinger you can direct as much of the dark area (areola) and nipple into his mouth as he can comfortably hold. He will receive your milk by compressing between his gums, tongue, and palate the middle and outer parts of the areola under which the milk ducts and small milk sacs are located. He will not get his milk as easily with only your nipple in his mouth and this hold would tend to make your nipples become sore.

Positions

Positions for nursing vary with each mother. The most important thing is to be comfortable so that you can relax completely. Some mothers prefer lying down, which has the practical advantage of providing a little rest as well. If you are about to feed your baby from your right breast, prop up your head, right shoulder, and upper back with a couple of pillows. Then lie your baby on his left side in the crook of your right arm. As you stroke his left cheek he will instinctively turn toward the breast, which you will help him take. In this position be especially careful not to let the breast you are feeding him with block his nasal passages. You can use your fingers to depress your breast next to his nose if this seems to be a problem, especially if your breasts are very full.

Some mothers prefer to sit when nursing their babies. A comfortable chair with supportive armrests and a footstool are helpful. You may find a rocking chair with comfortable armrests and back support suitable. A pillow in your lap may be handy for supporting your baby. Here again you may need to keep your thumb and forefinger on either side of the areola to keep his air passages open.

Supplementary Bottle

Let us suppose that in the hospital your baby was receiving both breasts and was apparently not getting enough milk. Your doctor may have decided that your baby needed formula in addition to your breast milk. You are going along with this, but are anxious about losing even more milk by substituting a formula. This concern is justified because milk production is stimulated in direct response to demand. In this event, you must deliberately cut down on the formula and count on your baby's increased hunger to give more stimulation to your breasts and thereby build up your breast-milk supply. This cutting down of the formula will probably make your baby hungry earlier. This becomes an example of demand feeding: You nurse him when he becomes hungry whether it is after four hours or even two hours. Your baby will indicate when his feeding is completed by turning his head, playing with the nipple, or falling asleep.

Your pediatrician may recommend that you give your baby a bottle once or twice a week even if your nursing is going along well. This is to ensure that your baby will take nourishment from a bottle in the event that it becomes necessary, and should not adversely affect your milk supply. Do not be surprised, however, if your baby balks at the bottle because formula is not nearly as tasty as mother's milk.

THE CASE FOR BOTTLE-FEEDING

There is nothing unnatural about a mother who either can't or won't breast-feed. The mother or father who bottle-feeds can hold the baby very close and become intimately acquainted with him. There are some advantages to bottle-feeding. If an infant is being bottle-fed, any member of the family or a baby-sitter can do the feeding. This allows the mother more freedom than if she were nursing. Father, in particular, can share in the feeding of his newborn, which can help alleviate his feelings of being "left out," and provide a warm bond between him and his baby. You may feel you can leave your baby more readily with your husband or sitter if he is conditioned to the bottle, which is true. You may also feel that breast-feeding will interfere with your time with your other children and bottle-feeding won't. On the other hand, you could reason that since breast-feeding does so much for the new baby in such a short time, you can spend time with your older child without fear of short-changing the baby. Some mothers worry about their older children being more disturbed by breast-feeding. Actually what disturbs an older child is any kind of close attention to the new baby. Ultimately, whether you breast-feed or not is in no way as important to your baby as a good start with his mother.

Although one may prepare formula using the specific milk and sugar proportions designated by a pediatrician, many parents today seem to prefer one of the commercially prepared formulas, selected with their pediatrician's approval. Commercially prepared formulas have a great many advantages: convenience, uniform composition, and controlled sterility and quality. (However, skim-milk formulas are considered inadequate and inadvisable for babies during their first year of life.) These formulas are available in ready-to-feed form and usually contain vitamins in amounts required by the baby. Of course, store-bought formulas are a little more expensive than homemade. All brands are basically the same. However, you need to prepare the formula exactly as indicated by the manufacturer. Too weak, the mixture will not provide sufficient nourishment; too strong, the mixture will have a concentration of possibly harmful mineral salts and excess calories. Remember to avoid formulas made with coconut oil because the latter is a highly saturated fat. In general, parents can feel confident when they use a formula recommended by their doctor. The Infant Formula Act gives the Food and Drug Administration the responsibility of making sure that all infant formulas have in them everything a baby needs.

Remember to hold the bottle so that the neck is always filled with milk. This keeps your baby from sucking in air, which could make him feel that his tummy is full before he has taken in enough milk. Some types of bottles have disposable liners that are designed to prevent air induction. You might want to try these and other types and decide for yourself.

Burp your baby at least once during the feeding and once afterward. If allowed to pass through his system, air bubbles can cause your baby pain. You can either place your baby on your shoulder and gently rub or pat his back, or sit him on your lap facing you while supporting his head with one hand and rubbing him on the back with the other. Some babies burp the minute they are straightened up; others need a lot of coaxing to bring up a bubble. The amount of bubbling, its frequency, and the position for bubbling should be determined individually. Protect your clothing with a diaper or a towel as some milk may come up right along with the bubble.

Hiccups are normal, being set off by bubbles returning. They often seem to clear up spontaneously, but can be stopped by putting the baby back to suck.

Checking the size of the nipple hole is probably the most important bottle-feeding basic because the flow of milk should correspond to the sucking-swallowing rhythm of the baby. The size of the nipple hole will determine how fast or how slowly the milk comes from the bottle. If the hole is too small, your baby will get air for all his sucking efforts. He may get tired before he gets enough milk and becomes uncomfortable or even throws up. He may also become colicky from all the air he has swallowed. If the hole is too large, the formula will come out too rapidly. This could cause indigestion or choking in extreme cases. It will also cut down on adequate sucking time.

Since your baby will know instinctively when he has had enough, be careful not to push him to finish his bottle. Your baby is the best judge of how much he needs at a particular feeding. Supplementing feedings with water, especially in hot weather, can calm a fussy, thirsty baby. After all, babies are not always hungry! As mentioned earlier, babies lengthen the intervals between feedings as they get older.

WARNING AGAINST FEEDING ENTIRELY ON DEMAND

Dr. T. Berry Brazelton cautions mothers against feeding a baby entirely on a demand basis. With a restless and fretful baby, it may lead to a great many feedings and consequently very little rest for the parents. In addition, it may encourage the baby to continue his night feedings indefinitely. However, if your baby is on the bottle, draining every one, and regularly waking early, your pediatrician should be consulted about increasing the formula.

If your baby wakes an hour or so after his last feeding, at which he finished his usual bottle, chances are against his being hungry so soon. Instead, it is more likely that he has been awakened by indigestion or colic. Try burping your baby again or seeing whether he will be comforted by some water.

Hunger is not always the reason your baby tries to eat his hand or takes the bottle eagerly. A colicky baby will indulge in both of these behaviors. It seems that the baby is unable to distinguish between colic pains and hunger pains. In other words, parents should not always feed a baby when he cries because it does not necessarily signify hunger. They need to study the situation and perhaps consult their pediatrician if the crying is unabated. Also, it makes sense to consider other possible causes first, and to change the baby's diaper, gently play with him, and check to see whether he is warm or cool enough. Only after ruling out such needs should feeding be tried. This approach helps babies learn that food is not the remedy for all ills.

SCHEDULED VERSUS DEMAND FEEDING

Each baby has his own internal time clock for hunger. Therefore, it is absurd to devise a fixed schedule, for example, an external time clock for all infants. Not only is each baby different from every other one, but even his hunger is likely to vary from day to day.

It took many years before doctors began experimenting with flexible schedules. In the early 1940s, Dr. P. McLendon and Mrs. F. P. Simsanian, a psychologist and a new parent, ran the first experiment on what they termed "self-demand feeding." They wanted to find out what kind of schedule a baby would establish if he were breast-fed whenever he seemed hungry. They found that in the first few days the baby woke rather infrequently. Then in the second half of the first week (just about the time the mother's milk began to come in), the baby awoke surprisingly often, about ten times a day. By the age of two weeks he had settled down to six or seven feedings a day, although they were at rather irregular intervals. Finally, by ten weeks the infant had arrived at approximately a four-hour schedule. Further investigation demonstrated that flexibility did not lead to diarrhea or indigestion, nor did it result in spoiling, as many had feared. On the contrary, many feeding problems were eliminated.

THE SCHEDULE IN THE HOSPITAL

Although many hospitals have incorporated the "rooming-in" plan and can accommodate the mother who prefers demand feeding, newborns are usually in a hospital nursery and fed by the clock. Full-sized babies are taken to the mother every four hours day and night, resulting in six feedings every twenty-four hours. Small babies are put temporarily on a three-hour schedule by day and a four-hour schedule at night, resulting in seven feedings in twenty-four hours.

THE SCHEDULE AT HOME

Babies tend gradually to lengthen the interval between feedings as they grow bigger. Because of the way a young baby's digestive system works, the average baby weighing six to nine pounds will last about four hours after an ample feeding at breast or bottle. It seems reasonable to suppose that with more frequent feedings, the baby would eat less each time, his stomach would empty more quickly, and emptiness would stimulate hunger sooner. Richard I. Feinbloom, M.D., of the Boston Children's Medical Center, suggests that the parent might try holding and rocking the baby or giving a few sips of water (not more than an ounce) to take the edge off the hunger. He believes that if the feeding could be held off for forty-five minutes to an hour, the baby would eat more, his stomach would then take longer to empty, and his hunger pangs would be postponed.

LATE-NIGHT FEEDING

The 10 P.M. or evening feeding is the one that mothers can most easily adjust to their own convenience. By the time the baby is a few weeks old, he is perfectly willing to wait for it until 11 P.M. or even midnight. The late-night feeding (2 A.M.) usually is given up by the end of the first or second month. One night when the baby is between two and six weeks old, he will sleep through until 3:00 A.M. or 3:30 A.M. This is to be treated as a 2 A.M. feeding. The next night he may sleep until 4:30 A.M. or 5 A.M. This should be counted as the 6 A.M. feeding, since the baby will generally not wake again until 10 A.M.

Pediatricians suggest that if the baby has reached the age of one month and weighs nine pounds and is still waking for a 2 A.M. feeding, the parents should try to give it up. They advise mothers not to let their babies sleep through the 10 P.M. or 11 P.M. feeding, even though the babies may be willing. Waking a baby at this time helps to avoid a feeding between midnight and 4 A.M. and tends to start the baby off somewhere between 5 A.M. and 6 A.M. each morning. When the baby is ready to give up one of his night feedings, the mother will want him to give up the 2 A.M. feeding first in order that her sleep will not be interrupted.

Bowel Movements

Your newborn's first bowel movement (referred to as passing *meconium*) will be thick and dark green or black. This substance filled his intestines before birth and must be expelled before normal digestion can take place. After that, the stools turn yellow-green.

The bowel movements of healthy babies vary in number, color, consistency, and general appearance. Breast-fed babies, for instance, have stools that resemble light mustard with seeded particles, and they may have a loose bowel movement after every feeding. The stools of formula-fed infants commonly are semisolid or solid, and tan or yellowish in color. If a baby's movements are always just a little loose, it can be ignored, provided he is comfortable, gaining weight, and the doctor finds nothing wrong.

Some babies normally have four to six movements a day. A baby is constipated only if the stools are hard and can be passed only with difficulty and bleeding. If your baby has such symptoms, discuss the condition with your doctor.

Diarrhea

Diarrhea in a baby under one year of age exists when he passes completely unformed or watery stools. Other signs of diarrhea include changes in color (from tan to green) and changes in odor. The stools may contain flecks of blood or mucus and be more frequent than usual. Sometimes a baby with severe diarrhea will pass as many as twenty or more stools a day.

Frequency of stools is the most important point to watch with respect to determining how severe an attack of diarrhea actually is. Doctors also are more concerned about changes in the consistency and odor of a baby's bowel movements than changes in the color of the stools. With mild diarrhea the stool changes are not very different from usual. Diarrhea in babies may also be accompanied by fever and vomiting.

If a breast-fed baby develops diarrhea, the first thing for the nursing mother to do is to check *her* diet and eliminate foods that might be causing the baby's diarrhea. Generally, this will clear up the problem. Diarrhea related to teething will be mild and stop as soon as the teething episode is over. Treating a baby with antibiotics for several days in the course of treating another condition may result in an attack of diarrhea. If this happens, you can easily remedy the situation by giving your baby either plain or flavored yogurt. Let your baby have as much as he wants two or three times a day, and be sure to check with your doctor.

Diarrhea due to formula, food intolerance, or food allergy

is treated by eliminating the offending substance, which is not always easy. Patience and persistence are often needed until the offending substance is identified.

Diarrhea due to infection generally is treated by a combination of medication and dietary restrictions. Most diarrheal infections in children improve after three to five days within the usual range of infections. Of course, how diarrhea is treated depends upon the cause and severity of the disorder. One general principle is to rest the baby's digestive system. You will know when your baby is getting better.

You may sometimes find the treatment of diarrhea hard to accept. For example, if your baby is crying for his bottle, it is hard to follow your doctor's orders only to moisten his lips with a wet cloth. Remember, however, that your baby cannot judge what is required in this situation. The best thing you can do for your baby is to follow your doctor's orders precisely. Better an unhappy baby for a while than a seriously sick one.

Vomiting

Many of us tend to confuse terms associated with vomiting. Here are definitions of these terms as they are used by health-care professionals:

1. Vomiting: stomach contents are returned accompanied by body spasms.
2. Projectile vomiting: vomiting so forceful that stomach contents will fly through the air and land a few feet away.
3. Spitting up: same as regurgitation; semidigested, curd-like milk just rolls out of the baby's mouth.

Now that we have defined the basic terms, let us discuss vomiting and some related conditions as they affect babies during the first year of life.

Hiccups are quite common in infancy. Causes include swallowing too fast, eating or drinking too much, or swallowing too much air along with a feeding. Hiccups generally do not last longer than five to ten minutes and usually stop without intervention.

Spitting up is another common occurrence in the early

months of life. It can be due to baby taking feedings too rapidly or in too great an amount. All infants spit up from time to time, even when they are perfectly healthy. The spitting up usually disappears when the baby is six months or so old.

Pyloric stenosis, an uncommon condition in which the valve (pylorus muscle) that leads from the far end of the stomach into the lower intestine does not open adequately to let milk pass through, is characterized by projectile vomiting after feedings. If this projectile vomiting occurs after more than two or three feedings or occurs once or twice a day for several days, contact your doctor. It is more prevalent in boys than in girls.

Feeding problems can cause vomiting. Overfeeding, not bubbling baby, too large holes in nipples, or a tense and anxious feeding situation can be involved. A good rule to remember is that vomiting related to feeding problems almost always occurs immediately *after* a feeding. Specific food allergies, as well as a formula that just does not agree with your baby, can also cause vomiting. Your doctor's guidance will be needed to pinpoint the exact cause and to remedy the condition.

Dehydration

The harmful effects of diarrhea and vomiting are almost entirely a result of excessive loss of water and salt from the body, which sometimes can be severe enough to cause dehydration. Dehydration occurs when fluid output exceeds fluid intake. Essentially, dehydration is corrected by treating the vomiting and/or diarrhea that caused it. If proper treatment is delayed, it can be very serious in babies. *If you suspect dehydration, contact your doctor at once.*

Signs of dehydration include infrequent urination, darker than usual urine, generalized weakness, listlessness, lethargy, an increased desire to sleep, and skin that feels dry to the touch. The baby's mouth will be dry also, his eyes sunken, and he will lose weight. Before a child becomes dehydrated there is a warning period when the loss of fluid is excessive in relation to fluid intake. Again, you must seek immediate medical help.

Sleep Patterns

All babies appear to possess an inner biological time clock. Since a great deal of a baby's first three months is devoted to sleeping, it is helpful for you to know what it is that your baby's built-in time clock is saying. Bear in mind, too, that your newborn will sleep only as much as he needs.

In a study conducted at the University of Toronto, the average newborn slept sixteen hours out of every twenty-four. Of course, the sixteen hours are only an average; babies (and adults) vary tremendously in their sleep patterns. Some infants spend eighteen hours or more sleeping, while other babies sleep as little as ten hours.

Newborn babies have several sleep cycles throughout the day, usually three to four hours in length. As infants grow older, their sleep requirements—in terms of cycles and hours—gradually decline. For example, by one month of age, most infants sleep only about fourteen hours out of every twenty-four. By one year of age, most babies have just two sleep cycles—the afternoon nap and nighttime sleep.

The sleeping behavior of infants will show the same characteristics as when they are awake. For example, an alert and noisy infant when awake will be active and noisy in his sleep. Each sleep cycle can be broken down into various types of sleep. At the midpoint of each cycle is a period of profound sleep with deep, regular breathing. The hour or so on either side of this deep sleep will be a lighter state in which movement and activity come and go. Breathing will alternate between shallow and deep. During this period there may be a drowsy, semialert state with irregular breathing at regular intervals, and the infant may make sucking movements with his mouth, move about, cry out, or just seem restless. Finally, the infant will either sleep again or waken fully.

Infant breathing patterns are often irregular. There may be periods of five to ten seconds when infants will stop breathing. This is known as an *apneic* spell. Normal infants outgrow this breathing pattern within the first few weeks of life. Actually, this particular kind of breathing is characteristic of a certain state of sleep. It appears to be a normal phenomenon in the newborn, and should not alarm parents unless it persists beyond the first few weeks. Talk to your pediatrician if you have any concerns about this.

Most newborns prefer to sleep on their tummies. It is fine to put your baby down in the position he prefers. Just be sure that your baby gets enough handling and changes of position and scenery when awake, and you really need not concern yourself with his sleeping position.

It is best not to bundle or swaddle your newborn while he sleeps. Light-weight covering to suit the season is best.

Cradles and bassinets make newborns feel especially secure, and many like to have their heads up against a bumper or other firm surface, which also helps them feel safe. You can give your baby this same feeling of security by placing him crosswise at one end of his crib. However, a baby should *not* have a pillow.

Ideally your baby should have a room of his own. Of course, a somewhat private area can work just as well. Do not stop making noise just because your newborn is sleeping. He will soon become accustomed to your usual household noises and sleep right through them.

A stressful situation may be created by the newborn who mixes up days and nights, for example, one who sleeps all day and then wakes up raring to go just when you are ready for bed. What can you do about this? Some parents keep their home as stimulating as possible during the day, with music, visitors, using infant seats and baby swings, and by waking the baby for feeding every four hours. At night, they reverse the schedule and decrease stimulation by darkening the baby's living area and responding to his needs in a calm, quiet manner.

Sometimes the above approaches do not work, and you may be faced with staying up and comforting a crying baby. Experienced parents offer these suggestions:

1. Sleep when your baby sleeps. Take enough naps so you get your normal quota of sleep.
2. Make yourself a pot of tea or whatever you prefer, find a comfortable chair for you and baby, put your feet up, turn on the television, and relax.

3. Remember that fortunately, this period will not last forever. Actually, many parents remember it somewhat fondly: Everyone else is sleeping; at this moment, the entire world consists of you and your baby. It is a perfect time to think beautiful thoughts about the present and the future.

For all newborns, there are time-tested sleeping aids. Playing a soothing music box, patting your baby's back gently as he lies in his bassinet, moving the cradle slowly and rhythmically, or rocking him while singing lullabies are some ways that help induce sleep. These measures have worked with generations of newborns and should work with your infant, too.

Your baby will have many more resources to assist him in falling asleep as he nears the end of his first year. The age-old comforting measures are especially valuable during the first three months, so use them to your baby's and your contentment.

Sedative-type medications should *not* be used to induce sleep in an infant unless a specific medical problem exists and your doctor prescribes one. If your baby does not sleep well, keep in mind that he will outgrow this as he matures. In the meantime, do what you can to alleviate his distress.

One of a Kind

Newborns are more powerful socially than previously believed. Your newborn is unaware that he exists. But he *is* an individual—with all the potential for impact that a real personality has on another human being. Every newborn varies infinitely from every other—in looks, feelings, movements, reactions to stimulation, and in his effect on his mother and father.

Babies are different even before their arrival. Some lie quietly in the womb, others allow their mothers little sleep in the last months before delivery. They "wake up" as mother prepares for bed and bicycle or kick for hours. Some infants are delivered from the womb screaming and fighting. Others appear sluggishly. Some newborns stay awake for as long as an hour and a half after birth before their first sleep. Others will fall into their deep sleep within a quarter of an hour after delivery. Boys in general differ from girls. They are more active, stronger, and less sensitive to pain.

Some newborns suck better than others. Some are alert longer and more frequently. Some prefer visual stimulation, others auditory. Some handle several kinds of stimulation simultaneously, others cannot. Some are more influenced by their needs for sleep, food, or physical comfort than others. Some are hard to arouse from deep sleep. Others will shoot directly from sleep to an inaccessible state of intense squalling. Some babies respond more vigorously than others to stimulation of all kinds. Some kick and flail as they become excited, while others become muscularly rigid. Some are "criers" right from the first day.

Many newborns can be soothed easily. Quieting others demands vigor. Some cannot be calmed with crooning, quiet rocking, or cuddling, or with a bottle or the breast alone. Tight swaddling, plus vigorous rocking, plus a bottle or the breast may do the trick. Do not feel awkward and unhappy if you have to quiet your baby this way. It may be the only thing that works. Many babies often behave like this and most do at certain times of the day. As Birns, Blank, and Bridger, researchers at Yeshiva University in New York City, have pointed out, the mother's and father's competence in protecting baby from their undue stress is what is important, not their way of doing it.

Other babies are so quiet and peaceful that new parents may worry about whether they are normal. They rarely cry, their color deepens slightly, and generally they respond almost imperceptibly to stimulation. They express disturbance subtly—a frown, a whimper, or sucking a finger or two. They may be limp and inactive for long periods. In contrast to a very active newborn who chokes down his formula with greedy, noisy gulps and then spits up some of it, this kind of baby feeds calmly and efficiently, bubbles quickly, and returns promptly to rest. Such neonates are not necessarily quiet because of the influence of their mother's sedation during delivery. They are quiet because it is part of their personality.

Scientists are conjecturing on the implications of the differences that appear at birth. A baby who cries no matter

Sudden Infant Death Syndrome

Sudden Infant Death Syndrome (SIDS), also known as crib death, causes the death of infants from one month to about four months of age. SIDS occurs to about one out of every 500 infants, usually between midnight and 6 A.M. The risk typically tapers off after six months.

The cause of SIDS is still unknown. The risk appears to be greater for male than female babies, and for black and Hispanic infants than for white babies. SIDS also seems to be greater among premature babies and those of low birth weight.

SIDS is the sudden, quiet death of an infant who has otherwise been basically well. Most of the babies die at home while they are asleep. There seems to be no single cause. In some cases, the death may be due to an abnormality in the baby's respiratory or cardiac systems or some deviation in his immune system. Close cardiac and respiratory monitoring is employed by the doctor in an attempt to circumvent the devastating death. Autopsies do not reveal an identifiable cause of these deaths.

The American Academy of Pediatrics recommends that healthy infants sleep on their backs or sides and not on their stomachs: Extensive research reviewed by an Academy task force shows a strong association between infants sleeping on their stomachs and SIDS.

According to Dr. Benjamin Spock, most babies not only prefer but insist on sleeping on their stomachs. He seeks more data before recommending a change in the sleeping position of babies. Other pediatricians maintain that infants generally do not have trouble adjusting to new sleep positions, and most parents will not face difficulties switching babies from stomach to back, especially in the newborn months.

Parents who lose their babies to SIDS usually find it impossible to avoid feeling guilty despite the fact that they could not have prevented their terrible loss.

how hard you try to calm him may evoke very different parental feelings than one who quiets within moments of soothing. Babies who respond to sights rather than sounds may fear strangers earlier and more severely. Newborns who are less affected by their internal needs may, as adults, be less hampered by their moods in working, thinking, and socializing. Newborns who rocket from one state to another without spending much time in between may convey their needs more clearly to their parents.

The reasons for newborn differences are a little clearer. Each baby starts life with a unique set of inherited characteristics—from each parent and from their families before them. Then, too, mother's diet, medication, personal habits, and general emotional health affect her newborn. So does the birth experience itself—the length of labor and type of delivery.

Besides, newborns are not really all the same age at birth. Age is counted from birth, but some babies have more developmental time in the womb than others. Premature babies may miss out on whole months of prenatal growth, and even some "full-term" babies are born a week or two before their due date. Others do not put in an appearance for as much as a week or two after they are expected. The baby lying next to yours in the hospital nursery and born on the

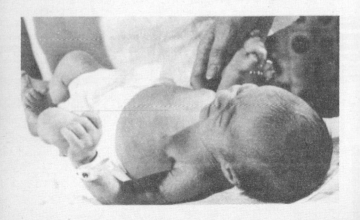

same date may thus be weeks older or younger. An "older" newborn is likely to be better developed, stronger, able to suck more vigorously, and less easily upset by sudden noises.

Whatever the implications or the causes of "difference," you can see from such variation that any description of the "normal" infant describes a statistical average, not any one baby. You should not expect such a profile to resemble your baby in all particulars. What it *can* do is give you some insight into the process of your baby's development—the way in which one kind of behavior leads to the next. The best way to understand your baby is to study the baby himself, learn his "cues," and respond to them appropriately. It is the little ways in which he differs from all others that makes him a special, interesting individual—*your* baby.

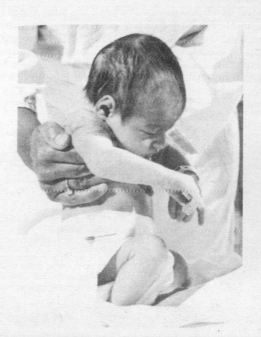

THE NEWBORN'S REFLEXES

If You	*Then the Baby's*
Tap bridge of baby's nose, shine a bright light suddenly into his eyes, or clap hands about eighteen inches from infant's head	Eyes close tightly (startle reflex).
Make sudden contact or noise	Head drops backward, neck extends, arms and legs fling outward and back sharply (Moro reflex).
Extend forearms at elbow	Arms flex briskly.
Lightly prick soles of feet	Knee and foot flex.
Stand infant; press foot to bed	Feet step.
Pull baby to sit	Eyes snap open, shoulders tense. Baby tries unsuccessfully to right head (china doll reflex).
Put baby on tummy on flat surface	Head turns to side and lifts. Baby crawls, lifts self with arms.
Support chest on water surface	Arms and legs "swim" (swimming reflex).
Place on back and turn head to side	Body arches away from face side; arm on face side extends, leg draws up; other arm flexes (tonic neck reflex).
Stroke foot or hand on top	Limb withdraws, arches, returns to grasp.
Stroke palm or sole at base of digits	Fingers or toes curl in (grasping reflex).
Stroke outside of sole	Toes spread, large toe sticks up (Babinski reflex).
Tap upper lip	Lips protrude.
Stroke cheek or mouth	Mouth roots, head turns, and tongue moves toward stroking object; mouth sucks (rooting reflex).
Stroke palm	Arm flexes; hand goes to mouth.

If You	Then the Baby's
Place object over nose and mouth	Mouth works vigorously; head twists, arms fling across face.
Stroke leg, upper part of body	Opposite leg or hand crosses to push your hand away; withdraws.
Rotate baby to side	Head turns, eyes precede direction of rotation.
Suspend by legs	Body curls to upside-down ball, legs extend, arms drop into straight line; neck arches backward.

THE FIRST WEEK

Motor Development	Language
### Gross Motor	### Vocalizing
Shows a variety of birth reflexes that are protective devices. (See prior listing of reflexes.) Some contribute to future physical development; others wither away.	Sounds are animal-like.
	### Responding
	Cries.
Reflexes control arm, leg, and hand movements. Non-reflexive activity is gross and random. Wiggles, kicks, flings arms and legs in all directions; twitches convulsively. Responds with total body to sudden changes.	
Moves head side to side, possibly up and down.	
When held on adult's shoulder, lifts head and adjusts posture.	
On tummy, lies in floppy, froglike position or rolled into ball.	
### Sitting	
Head falls backward or forward when pulled to sitting position.	
In prone position, with nose in mattress, can lift head high enough to prevent suffocation.	
Will startle if lowered through space rapidly, upon hearing a sharp sound, or when light is turned on.	
### Fine Motor	
Hands fisted. Reflex grasp.	
Reflex swallow. Eyes flair outward.	

Please do not regard this chart as a rigid timetable. Babies are unpredictable. Some perform an activity earlier or later than the chart indicates.

Mental	Social
### Sensory Response	### Personal

Mental

Sensory Response

Sees patterns, light and dark. Focuses eight inches in front of him; beyond that, vision hazy.

Sensitive to location of sound. Distinguishes volume, pitch; prefers high voice. Quiets when picked up or to any firm steady pressure.

Distinguishes tastes.

Attention Span

Alert about 3 percent of daylight hours.

Grips object if hand strikes it accidentally. Regards person momentarily.

Eye-Hand Coordination

Capable of tracking a small object touching mouth or lips (rooting behavior), and then sucking. Possesses simple reflexes; i.e., blinking eyelid when eyelid is touched.

When held, can track sound and moving object for short periods.

Body and Object Awareness

Stops sucking to look at something.

Discriminating and Associating

Shuts out disturbing stimuli.

Social

Personal

Shows excitement, distress.

Is individual in looks, feelings, activity level, and reactions to stimulation.

Interaction

Smiles spontaneously and fleetingly to sensory stimulation, like soft sounds.

Alerts to, tries particularly hard to focus on face or voice.

Quiets when picked up. Searches for breast.

Cultural Self-Help/Routines

Seven or eight daily feedings

Moves bowels often and sporadically.

Sleeps 80 percent of his day in five or six daily naps.

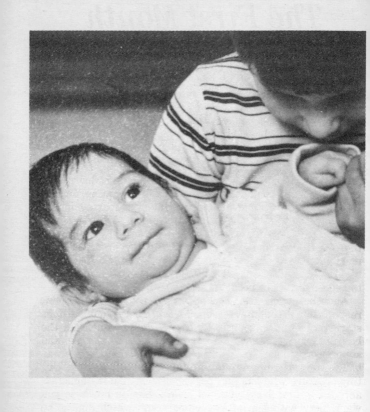

... spending as as before. They usually amuse you and please and want you to hold ... them. If you go to reach for them, they most likely react ... approval, and try to touch you back...

A very interesting turn about this ... ability that develops at this stage. Babies at this stage are ... their attention. The more things that seem also want to try and ... often uncontrollably. They want to ... it if they and better ... quickly if their attention is ... within their reach.

The First Month

FAMILY REORGANIZATION

The first month requires the reordering of baby's day and family life. From the moment of birth, he must learn new ways of getting food and oxygen and of eliminating wastes. His minimal practice with movement and hearing in the womb will amplify enormously in the outside world, while the seeing, tasting, and smelling that he could not practice there will start developing rapidly. In his first week, he must adjust not only to the world outside, he must also reorient himself from the bustling nursery at the hospital to the softer, more personalized atmosphere of home.

And there *you* are. The hospital routine and the joint responsibility that have helped you handle your feelings start vanishing as soon as the nurse helps you dress the baby in your room. She accompanies you to the car and almost ceremoniously resigns the baby to you and your husband, a ritual required by most hospitals. Suddenly, this tiny creature who has just begun to seem real is unmistakably *all yours!* Now you can cuddle him as much as you want, play with him after feedings, and watch him as he sleeps and wakes. With this new control, all your half-swallowed fears, doubts, and unsureness come to the surface.

A new mother who feels this overwhelming joy, responsibility, *and* anxiety is not alone. Every new mother experiences much the same thing. Many feel like weeping and often do—unaccountably. They wonder if they are inadequate or even if their uncontrollable feelings mean they are losing their minds.

Postpartum Blues

You may feel constantly drained. Everything requires more of you than it should and anything out of place provokes you to tears. If you do mobilize yourself to do something constructive, you are exhausted. If you cannot, you are annoyed with yourself. You know your husband would love some notice, but you can barely tolerate any affectionate overture. You feel alone, forsaken, and unwanted. If someone keeps you waiting for more than fifteen minutes, you think it is because you are the most unattractive, uninspiring female in the world. For the first time in your life, you feel like disagreeing with everyone. You call all your friends to come over and see the baby, although your doctor has warned you not to because of your fatigue and the risk of infecting the baby. Besides being somewhat depressed and bored, you may actually envy people. Any older woman's calm, experienced handling of the baby is threatening. You

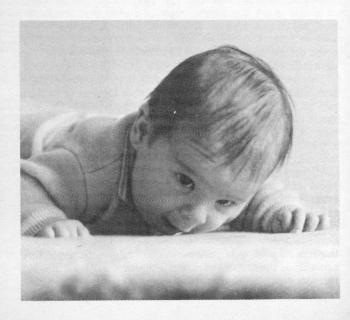

Some Mothers' Words on Postpartum Blues

"It is simply a release from the tension and excitement [of childbirth], a sort of cosmic anticlimax because your baby is not a Gerber Baby but a tiny (oh, how tiny!) wet, homely, demanding creature such as is never seen on commercials for baby food. Understand your disappointment and be assured it will pass."

"If you want to cry, cry! Everyone gets postpartum depression, so don't be concerned. It goes away."

"Talk about your feelings and keep on talking. Get as much sleep and rest as you can. When you are exhausted, everything is much worse."

"I didn't feel a depression, but I felt something—I call it 'postpartum weeping.' I wept with joy when I rocked the baby. I wept when Willie Mays played his last game. I know I am prone to sentimentality, but this was unbelievable."

contrast her competence with your confusion and helplessness and you wish you could just curl up in a ball in some quiet corner. The baby himself is frightening. He is so demanding with all his crying and seemingly endless eating.

The contrast between your possibly nightmarish fantasies and impatience with the baby and your dreams of being a perfect mother make you want to weep. So does your conviction that other young mothers are doing much better than you. A new mother's physical adjustment and recovery after delivery underlie this kind of behavior and emotion, which some people call postpartum blues.

Unfortunately, postpartum blues can be quite serious. More than fatigue and anxiety, it can be a real depression. It can come from hormonal changes that follow childbirth. (There are no conclusive research findings that offer specific medical explanations of how hormones affect emotions.) Some depression usually follows miscarriages or abortions; the loss of a baby is just too much to bear. Other factors can include the amount of stress in the new mother's life, her role expectations, exhaustion from the delivery, and such negative feelings as a sense of helplessness, discouragement, and insecurity. Depression can stem, too, from the mother's worrying about her infant's fragility, irregular breathing, and more. She may also become exasperated by her baby's crying and ceaseless needs. She may be concerned about her changed relationship with her husband.

Abnormal behavior can include rocking in a chair endlessly, refusing to feed the baby or to assume necessary chores. At the same time, some mothers become so engrossed in their feeding, bathing, and other routines that they fret about being left out of customary outside activities.

Postpartum depression, also called "childbirth psychosis," can continue for several months. If a mother's depression is profound, she should not hide it. Instead, she and her husband and their baby would all benefit if competent psychiatric help were sought early.

Maybe you will be one of the few lucky ones who more or less skips these blues. Their length will depend on your general physical and emotional health, the amount of support from your family, the difficulties of the birth, and your own drive. For some mothers, the very sight and sounds of home are enough to start their recovery. For others, the big adjustment taxes their physical and emotional reserves and often makes them unable to sleep and eat properly or to control their emotions.

Unfortunately, it's likely that the new mother's immediate family will be less helpful now than at other times. Her own mother may be suffering with her at long distance and her husband and children may increase their ordinary demands because of their own adjustment to the baby.

The two-year-old you are so eager to see again feels you have deserted him. His interest in the new baby is dutiful and he is terribly afraid you may leave him again. Even his father may seem to have abandoned him for the new intruder. He may be extraordinarily quiet and subdued, aggressive toward you and the baby, or incessantly demanding—showing off and dreaming up annoying mischief to distract you from his rival. His newly mastered toilet habits may disintegrate and he may insist on your feeding him all over again. If you can contain your surprise and shock at his antics, you may understand the reason for them

Where to Get Help for Postpartum Depression

1. Call the community mental health center for referral to a psychiatrist or other suitable agency. (Check your telephone yellow pages under "Clinics.")
2. Call your state Mental Health Division. Such divisions usually supervise mental health centers and make proper referrals upon request.
3. Write for information and referral to the National Institute of Mental Health Public Inquiries, 5600 Fishers Lane, Rockville, MD 20857.
4. Consult your own doctor.

As indicated earlier, the husband can also feel somewhat let down after the birth of his infant. His life has also changed remarkably. Both the mother and the father need to find some time to enjoy each other, in addition to their involvement with their baby.

and give him extra cuddling and comfort. Accepting his investigative intrusions with some good humor will probably help him satisfy his curiosity and minimize the chance of repeats. Shoving him away will only increase his feelings of exclusion, hurt, and jealousy.

An older child's reactions may be more complex than those of a two- or three-year-old. He may try to handle the family's changed relationships or your preoccupation by hardly noticing *you* at all, imitating you fiercely and mothering "his" or "her" baby whenever permitted. In a large family, he may wreak his real hostility on a younger child— stimulating him to be naughty and teasing him until he cries with frustration.

Your husband will be making his own adjustments. Secretly he is not at all sure what this new baby is going to do to his relationship with you. Modern American culture does not help a new father much, either. Although more hospitals are allowing the father to stay with his wife through labor, only a very few permit him to see his child born. After delivery, wife and child are unavailable to him.

He is allowed to see his wife only in prescribed, short doses of time so that she can rest and attend to their infant. A plate-glass window and hovering nurses keep him from his baby. The first time he really sees the newborn is when the nurse undresses the baby to put on his "going home" clothes.

FATHERING

More of today's new fathers are taking unpaid paternity leave, when they can, to share infant-care responsibilities with their wives, and to become more fully acquainted with their babies. Many fathers are moving from a left-out role to a co-parenting one.

Although the amount of time most fathers spend interacting with their infants is still small, research indicates that nurturing by fathers is on the rise in the United States.

Studies of father-infant attachment indicate that babies from around six months of age display attachment behaviors toward their fathers in pretty much the same manner as they do toward their mothers. Babies with fathers who helped care for them, played with them regularly, and were relatively patient with their fussing became attached to them early and intensely. Such babies smiled at, vocalized to, reached for, and tried hard to make physical contact with their fathers. Dr. Frank A. Pedersen, a research psychologist at the Social and Behavioral Sciences Branch of the National Institute of Child Health and Human Development, considers this attachment extremely valuable. He speculates that the father enhances his baby's independence by being interesting and desirable enough to draw the baby beyond the mother-infant duo.

According to Dr. Pedersen, some of the measurable positive effects on children when their fathers are nurturing include the development of their self-esteem, cognitive growth, active curiosity, social relatedness, and sexual identity.

In his book *The Nurturing Father*, Kyle D. Pruett, M.D., a child psychologist, presents the idea that men can directly involve themselves in raising their children with beneficial effects to themselves, their offspring, and the family unit.

"Men do not want to be baby-sitters nowadays; they want to be primary nurturing fathers."

It appears that fathers participate more in planning and providing child care when their wives work full- or part-time outside the home. However, caring for sick children continues to fall mostly on mothers or other consistent caregivers than on the average father.

In his book *The Birth of a Father,* Dr. Martin Greenberg, a psychiatrist, maintains that a father's positive feelings about parenting "help him weather the trials of the first year, and [enable him] to cope with his jealousy over his wife's preoccupation with their new baby." He believes that fathers also seek rewards, which may come in the form of pride about being a father and the ways in which their babies express their love for them.

Dr. Greenberg suggests that fathers who relish cuddling and playing with their babies need also to accept the grittier responsibilities—such as changing their infant's wet or soiled diapers. (Disposable diapers make the process more convenient!)

In *Dimensions of Fatherhood,* Shirley M. H. Hanson and Frederick W. Bozett write: "Infants are able to distinguish fathers from other adults very early. In turn, fathers interact with them in somewhat different ways than mothers. They tend toward more rough and tumble play." Actually, the quality of time spent with one's child may be as important as the amount of time. A baby can absorb a great deal of his father in a very short time. Both benefit immeasurably from their shared experiences.

It has been clearly established and much documented that father-absent or father-weak homes may result in boys who identify too closely with their mothers, or who will show overly aggressive behavior; for instance, as seen in juvenile delinquents. The current phenomenon of the absent father is particularly hurtful to little boys. Of course, little girls are also deprived when they are denied sensitive fathering. Both same-sex and opposite-sex parents are vital to their children's well-being.

Yet the finding that fathers have the potential to be competent at child care does not mean that all fathers will be capable or will enjoy child care. The same may be said of mothers. In addition, not all children are uniformly easy to rear.

GRANDMOTHERS CAN HELP, TOO

During these first weeks at home grandmother can be a real help. Her main assets are her moral support for mother and her experience as a mother. In addition, she may assist with baby care, housekeeping, even in alleviating father's tension, depending on her relationship with him.

Her role is not easy. Besides her own conflict between needing to be with you and wanting to be at home, she may often face your very natural jealousy. She is a "fair" target for anger, defensiveness, and frustration, while she herself may be struggling to keep her promises to stay in the background and restrain the very human need to give sound advice. She might return home at the end of her stay feeling that she has failed to help you relieve your tension. Yet she can give you and your husband time—time to get yourselves together to mother and father your baby. Nobody can do your job for you. But depending on her tact in presenting her ideas, some of them may get through and help you in her absence.

Creature of Habit?

The baby must also adapt dramatically. Life in the hospital's newborn nursery is a far cry from a quiet room in a home's nurturing world. He has learned how to defend himself against intense light, the constant noise of busy nurses and screaming infants, and the physical discomfort of impersonal, sometimes rough handling, and of being wet, dirty, and hungry at times that did not fit the schedule of a hospital staff.

For some days after you bring him home, your baby will be a very disorganized little fellow. Most newborns are active at birth, quiet for the next few days, then more active again the first days at home. They cry a lot and eat poorly, frequently, and erratically. If your baby is breast-feeding, he may suck for long stretches of thirty to forty minutes at each breast on some days, but only ten to twenty minutes on others. He probably won't quiet with handling as well as he will later. He wakes fitfully, breathes irregularly, sneezes, chokes, spits up, vomits occasionally, and startles frequently.

According to Dr. Peter H. Wolff, a neurophysiologist at the Massachusetts Institute of Technology, a month-old baby sleeps more than he does anything else, cries more than he is active, and divides the small time he is awake between drowsiness and alertness. He sleeps much more than you do, at least twelve and usually about fourteen hours. While his eyes may be shut for more than that, he will actually be awake and can receive and respond to stimulation.

He also sleeps differently from you. You have only two sleep phases; the baby has three, though his sleep phases do not differ as sharply as yours. His sleep may be light or restless, periodic, or deep. His deep sleep features no activity, a reposed face, regular breathing, firmly closed eyelids, and little response to stimulation.

Neonates are mostly light sleepers. Scientists know this because they have recorded the distinctive brain wave pattern and greater body movement associated with dreaming. At birth about half your baby's sleep is restless and 20 to 30 percent is deep. His level of sleep fluctuates according to an internal clock. He may rouse in regular three-hour cycles, or cry out more sporadically, raise his head, move to the top of the crib, and quiet. Almost all of his deep sleep episodes are about twenty minutes long. By about the second week, this timing is so regular that you can predict when your baby will wake or become restless. Gradually this whole pattern reverses itself so that the eight-month-old approximates the adult's sleep pattern of 50 to 70 percent deep sleep and 20 to 25 percent dream time.

When your baby is sleeping lightly, he is more susceptible to inner and outer stimulation, and you can see all kinds of behavior. He whimpers, grimaces, smiles, sneers, frowns, pouts, mouths rhythmically, breathes irregularly, and if you watch very closely, you can see his eyes darting beneath the lids. Sleep smiles are different from the social ones you will see a bit later when your baby's eyes are bright and

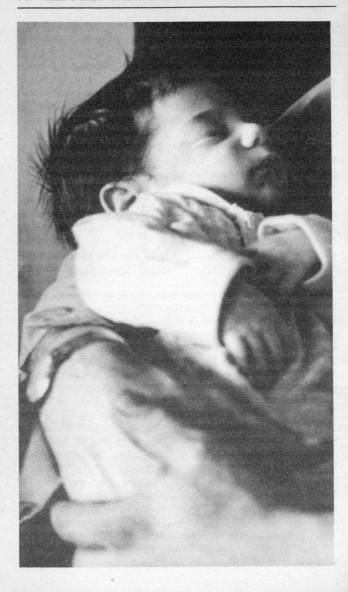

his whole face lights up to a voice or a face. A sleep smile, which is often stimulated by sounds, just works the muscles of his lower face.

Newborns also catnap, rather than sleep in long stretches. The longest newborn sleep period is about four to five hours. Usually seven or eight naps alternate with wakeful states ranging from a drowsiness that looks like drugged stupor to wild flailing of arms and legs and frantic crying.

A baby can actively squirm, kick, or suck on his fist as much as twelve hours a day. A few causes of his increased activity are fairly apparent. A baby grows more active before feeding and urination. He also becomes very overwhelmed by pain or other disturbing outside stimulation and sometimes sets up a cycle of activity that only you can interrupt. His activity upsets him and further sensitizes him to the offensive stimulation. The more sensitive he becomes, the more vigorously he struggles. Some bursts of activity seem triggered by fatigue, long periods of lying awake, or looking around.

Some psychological causes also seem at work. Loosely wrapped swaddling can rouse a baby to outrage even though it is not painful, while he calms down when well swaddled.

While all this activity may look pointless to you, it is very important to your baby's growth. These basic movements will later differentiate and become coordinated with the baby's reflexes to become part of his developing motor patterns.

Why Do Babies Cry?

Crying and fretting often go with your baby's thrashing about—a combination he is most likely to break into if he is hungry, thirsty, tired, or frustrated. Crying is really his first social communication. It is not terribly sophisticated but it is useful. Partly because it is a distress signal of children and adults, partly because it is irritating, partly because of instinct, mother usually comes running to discover what is making her baby cry.

On some days your baby may cry for twenty to thirty minutes four or five times a day before feedings, sleeping, or elimination. You can modify this before naps by placing your baby on his tummy. This position helps him control the startling that still accompanies his crying. On other days the baby's crying, squirming, and fussing before sleeping in the evening can last from one to three hours at a time. The longer periods may follow a noisy, busy day, a weekend when father is at home, or a "blue period" for mother.

After lying for hours looking around quietly, he may slowly begin whimpering. At first he can be talked to and will become alert and stare at your face for several minutes. You can rock him for almost thirty minutes before he tires and begins to wail again. But sooner or later he will reach a point when no comforting really succeeds more than briefly. Play, rocking, swaddling, changing his diapers, and feeding him to be sure he isn't hungry are all useless. He will continue to cry for long stretches, tapering off to deep, shuddering sobs before sleep. These periods may be his attempts to discharge enough energy so that he can settle down. Infants who fuss are more likely to sleep for long periods at night.

This timing at day's end is not entirely haphazard. Dr. Anna Freud writes of the falling to pieces of a baby's ego at the end of a day. The family's fatigue, the mother's own ego disintegration, and the expectant excitement around a father's homecoming all contribute.

Exercising Your Baby

According to Suzy Prudden and Jeffrey Sussman in their book *Suzy Prudden's Creative Fitness for Baby and Child*, an infant can be gently and playfully exercised at six or seven days of life and thereafter. For example, you can take your baby's tiny hands in yours and carefully unfold his arms so they are outstretched toward you. Then fold them back, unfold them to the side, and fold them back up to his shoulders. Repeat a few times if your baby appears to be having fun. After you exercise your infant's arms, hold his ankles and gently straighten his legs and then fold them. Repeat smoothly a few times.

Studies on infant crying show that environmental tension does add to the length and intensity of crying spells. A baby can tune in his family's feelings. When his mother is tired or tense, he is impossibly fussy. When she is rested and unharried, he is delightfully responsive. Studies show that crying for "unknown causes" decreases sharply when a baby gets more nurturing—handling, talking to, looking, and listening.

Do not feel badly if you cannot soothe your baby as quickly or easily as you expect. There may be nothing wrong with either you or him. Some crying may simply be inevitable and necessary. Psychologists tell us a "bad" day of crying and fussing may indicate tension before a thrust into a new developmental stage. The good, quiet, peaceful days are usually those when your baby is operating on the same level and not responding to any kind of change. The ability of parents to protect their infant from undue stress as well as the infant's ability to respond to various soothing techniques may strongly affect the relationship between parents and child.

SOOTHING TECHNIQUES

The techniques for soothing a crying baby are as numerous as there are mothers, fathers, and babies. Holding, rocking, patting, and softly singing are, of course, the old reliables.

Soothing techniques are important tools in coping with a crying infant. With knowledge of the approaches generally acceptable to infants, and sensitivity to which of these are most effective in dealing with *your* baby, frustration triggered by prolonged crying can be avoided.

Swaddling is one of the oldest forms of soothing a very young crying baby. Simply placing a baby's arms by his sides and wrapping him snugly in a blanket will often be enough to interrupt the continual startle reaction (the Moro reflex) that otherwise can keep him crying for prolonged periods. Please note that many doctors question whether a baby should be swaddled routinely inasmuch as restricting the free movement of his arms and legs may retard his physical development.

Picking up a crying infant and putting him to the shoulder

is a soothing technique that often induces a state of alertness that may be optimal for the infant's earliest learning. Because a picked-up infant frequently becomes visually alert and scans the environment, he will have more opportunities to learn about his environment than a baby left crying in the crib. Since early stimulation appears necessary for normal human development, the visual experiences given to a crying infant when he is picked up may be an important by-product of this soothing technique.

Dr. Spock believes that such comforters as a cuddly toy, a piece of cloth, a bottle, a pacifier, or a thumb are soothing to infants and children at different ages for various reasons. Usually thumb- or pacifier-sucking in the first six months merely expresses a baby's need to suck. There is no reason to either encourage or discourage this behavior in infants.

Babies tend to form attachments on the basis of the kind of stimulation they want and get. A baby may prefer the uncle who rocks him to the one who tickles, just as he may prefer one voice to another. You might work out a system of letting him cry for a while, then picking him up and cuddling him, getting bubbles up, and putting him back to bed. Handling him calmly with this routine may quiet him.

Furthermore, some babies soothe more easily than others; for instance, an infant easily soothed by one stimulus tends to be easily soothed by all stimuli, and a baby unresponsive to one approach is difficult to soothe with any other.

Of course, babies differ in the amount of crying they seem to need, depending upon physical and emotional factors that are not always easily understood. Nothing deflates a parent's self-confidence more than not being able to comfort and silence a crying infant. Of course, crying is the baby's way of communicating various needs and feelings. Parents learn to discern the messages delineated by the different pitches, intensities, and urgencies of their offspring's crying. Stoicism, patience, and experience have long mileage in caring for a crying infant. However, do take heart! All babies do some crying, and few are "crybabies" when they attend nursery school. Experience enables a mother and a father to learn what approach works best with their baby.

Some doctors find that babies held in close contact over

their mothers' hearts cry less. The heartbeat seems to soothe them, possibly because in the womb each heard his mother's heart. The late Dr. Lee Salk of the New York Hospital-Cornell Medical Center had some fascinating things to say about this. Babies respond to music as early as the first month, probably because the tempo of music, from the most primitive to the most modern, is usually between fifty and one hundred and fifty beats per minute, essentially the range of the human heartbeat. Most mothers, both right- and left-handed, do in fact hold their babies on their left side, including mothers in sculpture and paintings from Italian Renaissance to Henry Moore and Picasso.

Alertness

The one-month-old is alert only a small portion of the time he is awake. Dr. Wolff clocked about three hours of intermittent alertness from about thirty hours of wakefulness a week. This is your baby's natural playtime, the best time for a little sociability, a little getting to know each other. The baby can lie quietly on his back, alert and listening, for as much as an hour or as little as a couple of minutes half a dozen times a day. He will quiet more readily and be more responsive to novel sights, sounds, and stimulation after a changing, feeding, and bubbling than before, when hunger and other physical discomforts interfere.

Since the first increases in the length of your baby's alertness occur only when he is comfortable, relieving these irritations is most important. Short as they are, your baby's alert periods are prerequisites for more advanced learning. As Dr. Howard A. Moss of the National Institute of Mental Health says, "The amount of time an infant spends at a given level of consciousness is clearly going to influence the way he experiences the world, the types of discriminations he makes, and his level of mental organization." For example, the important ability to follow and observe something carefully develops primarily when your baby is alert.

Some investigators have even speculated that visual stimulation in the first four months facilitates the growth of the visual apparatus. A stimulating environment allows the month-old baby to organize his responses to external events

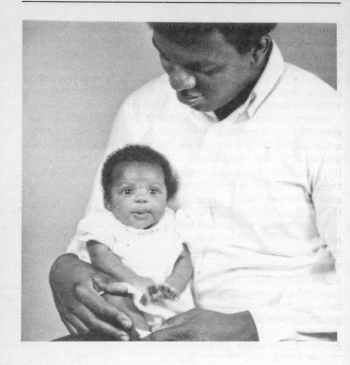

rather than just his physical needs. His attention to an interesting taste, smell, sight, or sound actually controls diffuse, aimless activity. When the eyelids of a drowsy baby finally close, spontaneous energy discharges occur that seem inhibited as long as his eyes are open.

Since the baby's alertness is apt to evaporate as soon as an interesting spectacle is removed, you can keep him alert by focusing his attention on an interesting sight, such as a moving toy or a mobile, or a sound, perhaps a bell toy. In fact, for a tiny baby just as for us, meaningful encounters with the environment are one critical way to maintain alertness. Dr. Wolff found that a provocative, interesting environment may alert even a fussy or drowsy baby. Even if it does not, as long as his lids remain open, a drowsy baby appears to register his sight experiences, which seem to impress him. There may be a whole range of seemingly meaningless stimuli that, despite the baby's apparent indifference, contribute to his learning and behavior. After all, you can read a book or watch a movie without indicating to anyone what you have learned and without changing your visible behavior in any way.

Babies seem to *choose* to stay awake for stimulation and activity. Once they have been fed and their physical comfort attended to, they certainly do not need to stay awake. All *you* need to know is how much sleep, stimulation, and activity your baby seems to need. Babies are individualists in these matters as in everything else. You will soon find what amount of excitation your baby can cope with, as well as the method of soothing that your baby responds to best.

If you are in touch with your baby, you will respond to his preferences. When he is tense and highly aroused, you may soothe him. When he is quiet and alert, you can play with, talk to, and show him things because it pleases both you and the baby. The important point is that if a baby's tensions are relieved as they arise, he soon gets the idea that the world is a good place, and the people in it worth getting to know.

Some Common Occurrences

COLIC

Colic, a catchall term used to explain almost any hard, persistent crying, is unfortunately a common disturbance in infancy. It seems that as many as 80 percent of babies are afflicted even when they are completely healthy. Colic may begin anytime between the second and fourth week, but gradually disappears by the time the baby is three months old. Due to the regularity of the pattern, it is commonly known as "three-month colic."

During a classic colic seizure, a baby will stir uncomfortably soon after the early evening feeding, or even before it is finished, and shriek for three or four hours with hardly any respite. Neither rocking, burping, a pacifier, nor a drink of water will calm a colicky infant. At 10 or 11 P.M. the baby may fall asleep, possibly after having downed the 10 P.M. bottle. The next morning the baby is contented and feeding well, only to repeat the nerve-shattering performance at 6 P.M. It is characteristic of colicky babies that they seem to thrive well and suffer no permanent impairment, but the wear and tear on their parents is horrendous.

Whereas one baby may be very regular about his colic attack, always complaining between 6 P.M. and 10 P.M. or 2 P.M. and 6 P.M., another baby may cry over a longer period of time. The latter may be peaceful in the evening but disturbed on and off throughout the day. Most upsetting to parents, of course, is the baby who sleeps all day and wails half the night. The baby who starts out being restless during the day and then gradually shifts to the night, or vice versa, is also a torment to his parents.

Very young infants are especially prone to the swallowing of air. If the bubble is not brought up and passes down into the baby's intestine, colic can result. The sporadic spasms of colic occur because the intestinal muscles contract sharply in trying to move the bubble on. Colic may be suspected when the infant draws his legs up sharply with each spasm of pain.

Babies who cry frantically tend to draw in large amounts of air (and consequently their abdomens become distended with gas), and they may pass gas via the rectum. Colic can be a baby's response to overfeeding, underfeeding, a milk allergy, an infection, intestinal complaints, or just being a terribly fussy infant.

When a baby turns colicky, the mother's first reaction is to suspect the feedings. Crying from colic usually begins *after* feeding and in this way can be distinguished from hunger cries, which usually occur *before* feeding. Most mothers instinctively want to feed a baby who is crying, but this is not advisable in the case of a colicky baby. The problem does not appear to be related to food, because colic may occur with feedings of breast milk and all kinds of formulas.

Some infants do not tolerate certain foods in the nursing mother's diet, mostly certain fruits and vegetables. Garlic and onions may cause colic in some infants, while cabbage, turnips, broccoli, or beans may make others gassy and colicky for hours. The same has been said of rhubarb, apricots, and prunes. Melons, peaches, and other fresh fruits may also cause diarrhea and colic in infants. If your baby is bottle-fed, a change of formula occasionally helps.

Mothers are warned that crying may result if the baby is swallowing too much air while nursing. Such crying, unlike colic, may be eliminated by holding the baby with his head higher than his tummy during feeding. Research indicates that the mother's temperament, anxiety level, and degree of success in adapting to the maternal role are *not* factors in the development of colic. More research is needed to discover the exact origin of colic.

You can try to soothe your baby with cuddling; soft, loving words; gentle rocking; pacing the floor; and so on. There are no guarantees in treating colic, and the knowledge that most babies get over it by three months of age does not help distraught parents. Some relief may be derived from laying your colicky infant on his tummy across your legs while you gently pat or massage his upper back. Try to alternate your baby's night care, and take occasional nights off to help restore your frayed nerves and battered ears, even if this means just getting out of the house and going for a walk.

Have your pediatrician examine your baby to find out if a specific problem exists. Fortunately, colic does not appear to do babies any permanent harm.

DIAPER RASH

Your baby may develop a diaper rash no matter how careful you are. The most common causes of diaper rash are tightly fitting diapers; too much ammonia in your baby's urine (a normal waste product in many infants); infection due to bacteria or yeast; an allergic reaction to something your baby breathes or eats; and irritating soaps or detergents.

Change your baby's diaper as soon as possible after a bowel movement. Wash the area with a soft cloth and water. Also change wet diapers frequently to reduce skin exposure to moisture. If the baby's skin is dry, use a soothing baby lotion or ointment. If the rash is moist, use a baby drying lotion or salve.

Mild rashes usually respond to more frequent diaper changes and the use of a protective coating (zinc oxide ointment, for one). If your baby's diaper rash lingers for more than three days, consult your doctor.

PRICKLY HEAT

Babies develop prickly heat when they are hot and sweating. Usually found around the neck and shoulders, it appears as clusters of raised pink splotches with white centers. The treatment is to apply a thin coating of a cornstarch powder and to dress the baby coolly. Put the powder in your hand and then gently pat it on so your baby will not breathe any of it into his lungs.

THUMB-SUCKING

Thumb-sucking is misconstrued as a problem; actually it is a normal reflex. In a study by Harvard's Pediatrics Department, 86 percent of the observed healthy and apparently normal babies showed that they enjoyed sucking their thumbs even though they were not fatigued, hungry, or uncomfortable. The investigation indicated that finger- or thumb-sucking began between birth and three months, gradually increased in intensity to a peak by seven months, and then decreased as motor development occupied the baby more. This same period marks the onset of mouthing objects and most likely contributes to the decline of thumb-sucking. By twelve months, except during periods of stress or tension, most of the babies had ceased to suck their thumbs.

A breast-fed baby is less apt to be a thumb-sucker because the mother is more inclined to let the infant continue nursing for as long as he wants to. Since it is impossible for the mother to know when her breasts are empty, she has to rely on her baby. Although the baby gets most milk from the breast within five or six minutes, he may be eager to continue sucking for as long as thirty minutes to satisfy the craving to suck.

On the other hand, when the baby finishes a bottle, it is done. The infant is forced to stop because sucking air is unpleasant. Therefore, thumb-sucking is likely to begin at about the time the baby learns to finish the bottle in ten minutes instead of twenty. This happens because the baby is getting older and stronger and the rubber nipples are getting weaker. One possible solution is to buy new nipples.

THUMB-SUCKING AND TEETHING

Quite commonly around the age of three to four months the baby may begin to chew on thumb and fingers. The tendency to extend the arms, especially as the head is turned, gives way to ease of flexion at sixteen weeks, thus allowing babies to put fingers or thumbs into their mouths more easily. This may be due to teething and should not be confused with thumb-sucking per se. During teething periods, the baby who is a thumb-sucker is sucking one minute and chewing another.

In addition to being related to feeding behavior, thumb-sucking often is associated with sleep. Many babies suck their thumbs or fingers to comfort themselves as they fall asleep, which is quite natural.

Many parents worry about the effect of thumb-sucking on their baby's teeth and jaws. Dentists indicate that any tilting of the baby teeth has absolutely no effect on the permanent teeth that begin to come in at about six years of age. In other words, if thumb-sucking is given up by six years of age, and in the majority of instances it is given up by four or five, there is little chance of its affecting the permanent teeth.

Generally, it is agreed that using any type of restraint, such as elbow splints or mittens, is a bad idea. Similarly, scolding a baby makes no sense. It would only make the baby miserable, frustrate him, and tend to prolong the habit.

Progress Report

The drama of a new baby's homecoming and the upheaval of all the principals around him are by no means exaggerated. The first three weeks of life away from the hospital are probably the longest and most depleting of a family's relationship with its newest member. Most families suffer disruption as everyone regroups toward the goal of being a

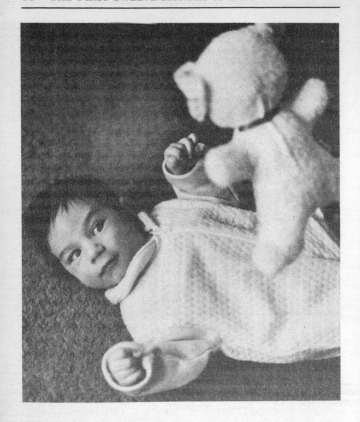

bigger-by-one family. But gradually you will regain your physical and emotional strength. Your first-week slump may even be a necessary part of adapting to motherhood. Even the baby, although he still seems to spend a lot of time sleeping, has been busy every moment adjusting to life on the outside. He has had lots of new jobs to do simultaneously and you will probably have noted many changes.

He is heavier than he was when he was born, although he only regained his birth weight somewhere around the tenth day of life.

He is still a little bundle of reflexes, but he's not so limp anymore. This is partly because the brain itself is firmer and less gelatinous. His muscles are firmer. Millions and millions of new connections have grown between millions and millions of nerve cells in his organs, as well as his muscles.

His eyes do not seem to roll around in his head so much; the twelve tiny muscles controlling them are better organized, and he is learning to control them and to focus his eyes a little more quickly and often. He tries so hard to focus, particularly to a face or toward a voice, that his eyes sometimes cross, his body shivers, and he begins to hiccup with the effort. He is beginning to "reach" with his eyes.

He breathes more regularly, and chokes, vomits, trembles, and startles less. In a few weeks, his spontaneous startles during sleep will have been reduced to occasional twitches in his face, hands, and feet.

Instead of total unpredictableness, he may now move his bowels only once, but probably no more than four times a day on waking from sleep.

Feeding and Sleeping Patterns

Waking and sleeping states differ more clearly with fewer gradations between. A primitive pattern sets in. The baby wakes most when he is hungry, then cries, feeds, becomes alert, grows drowsy, and sleeps again.

Other patterns are beginning to stabilize more and more. By the third to fifth week, your baby may reduce his seven or eight feedings to five or six over a twenty-four-hour day, with four-hour stretches between feedings during the day.

From seven or eight periods of sleep in every twenty-four hours, he has probably reduced the daily naps to three or four and combined two of them into one five- or six-hour nighttime sleep, possibly after the 10 P.M. feeding. He is establishing a simple cycle of quiet and unquiet, night and day. By two weeks he takes as much as eighteen ounces of milk daily, increasing to twenty-four or twenty-five ounces by four weeks.

In contrast to the excessive crying and accompanying uncoordinated movements of the first ten days or so of life, his total crying time may begin to decrease as you handle him with more understanding and less anxiety. His interested, alert periods will lengthen. He has learned to mouth his fist or suck his thumb and can shorten the crying and fussing himself. As time goes on, he may differentiate the first two fingers of one hand and learn to suck on them with loud smacks of comfort. After his explosive bouts, he seems to eat and sleep better.

Well-Baby Checkups

The best way to make sure your baby is thriving is to have him checked regularly by a pediatrician. Monthly visits are recommended for the first six months. For the second six months, monthly or bi-monthly visits are in order.

The most important friend a baby and his parents have is the doctor. Regular visits to his or her office are enlightening and helpful. They offer parents a routine source of information and security, and enable them to relieve themselves of worries that may have been building up during the month. It is a good idea to keep a notebook handy for recording questions as they arise, and for indicating new developments.

At the same time as the physician builds a medical picture of your baby, his or her guidance and opinion may be elicited on various aspects of childrearing that go beyond medical considerations. For example, the parents of a firstborn might be anxious about what is actually perfectly normal behavior. The pediatrician can easily pick this up and reassure them. Also, on the basis of rather diverse and mild symptoms, the doctor may recognize an "allergic-type" baby at a very young age, and suggest that the parents introduce new foods very cautiously and make every effort to control other irritating factors in the baby's environment.

The baby—the "star" member in the cast—reaps many benefits from this ongoing relationship. Babies are not born afraid of doctors; in fact, they may be fascinated by them at first. When they are quite young, a trip to the doctor's office means many new and interesting things to see, hear, and touch. Nevertheless, a baby learns very quickly to be

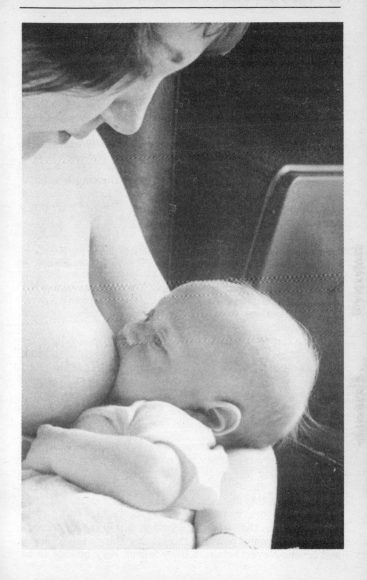

When to Call the Doctor

There comes that inevitable time when your baby's appearance, disposition, and/or general behavior seem different to you. You are faced with the problem of whether or not to call the doctor. When in doubt, the rule is to call. The doctor, with his or her vast experience over a period of time with a large number of babies and their parents, can answer your questions until you are completely satisfied.

Below is a list of symptoms that should be reported to your doctor:

1. Your baby looks or acts differently (unusually pale, tired, listless, irritable, restless).

2. Your baby has a fever of 101°F. (Remember, however, that babies can be quite sick yet have no fever.)

3. Colds: if they get worse, if there are any new symptoms, if your baby looks sicker.

4. Hoarseness, difficulty in breathing: report at once.

5. Pain in ears, stomach, urinary tract. (Headaches in a small child should be reported.)

6. Sudden decrease in appetite. If this occurs with other symptoms, call your doctor at once.

7. Vomiting: report promptly; also diarrhea.

8. Blood in stools or vomitus.

9. Inflammation of the eye.

10. Injury to the head: report in 15 minutes if your baby is not reacting normally.

11. Bulging of the soft spot (fontanel).

12. Injury to a limb: if your baby is not using it or shows pain on using it.

13. Burns: report if blisters appear.

14. Poisons.

15. Cuts.

16. Nosebleeds.

17. Rashes: most common is diaper rash in the first year. Most contagious diseases are not applicable to the first half year of life. If your baby seems sick with a rash or the rash is extensive, call the doctor.

Some Safety Tips

Make sure you have a safe crib, infant seat, and high chair.

Never use a plastic cover on the crib mattress.

Remember to keep the crib sides up and do not use a pillow.

Never leave your baby alone on a bath table or any surface other than an uncluttered floor.

Strap your baby in securely when he is in an infant seat, high chair, or car restraint.

Always check the bath water before you put in your baby, and never leave him alone in the bath, not even for a minute.

Put in electric plug guards even before your baby begins to crawl.

Small objects, medicines, soaps, assorted pins, powders, vitamins, oils, cleaning substances, and all plants should never be within your baby's reach.

apprehensive when the doctor starts to do unpleasant things to him. Strange instruments are stuck into his ears, nose, and mouth; needles are injected; the poking and probing of his whole body are hardly enjoyable. Parents need to be sympathetic to the cries of discomfort that their baby expresses while they communicate the need for the checkups.

A baby up to about one and a half years old cannot be prepared for a visit to the doctor. Unable to understand the doctor's function, he reacts to what is done to him. If it is pleasant, he likes it; if it is unpleasant, he dislikes it. Parents should hold and cuddle their baby when he is unhappy, talk to him, and sympathize with him. Whenever possible, distraction is a helpful device.

To sum up, regular, thorough checkups by a competent, friendly pediatrician may be described as "preventive medicine in action." Choose a doctor you can talk to: one who will be helpful in allaying your concerns. In addition to a careful physical examination of the child, the pediatrician needs to directly assess the child's coordination, behavior, and so on. Ideally a regular checkup permits the pediatrician and the parents to compare notes and to check out any difficulties that might impede the healthy growth of the child. First-time mothers and fathers need all the support they can get.

Always check with your pediatrician for the latest medical information available relative to your baby's health and well-being.

By now you are quite good at understanding his different cries of hunger, discomfort, pain, or boredom. You will also recognize some new sounds—throaty noises called cooing.

Another emotion is emerging—enjoyment. He cries when wet and quiets when changed. He enjoys his bath, probably because of the handling involved.

A new kind of crying just before he falls asleep signals a new stage of development, a readiness for experiences. He wants to be held, carried, or propped so he can look around.

You may also notice that his fixed staring at things—sometimes as long as ten to fifteen minutes—is followed by a new kind of behavior. He becomes excited when he sees a person or a toy. He moves his arms and legs, pants, vocalizes, and even smiles, with a kind of readiness to respond.

A baby does not yet distinguish between his actions and their results. The world is hungry, or warm, or wet, or feels good. Things just seem to appear and disappear before the new infant, as though he were seeing them, according to the late Dr. Jean Piaget, through the window of a moving train. But by four weeks, he will begin to repeat actions for their own sake; for instance, kicking for the pleasure of it.

Although there is still no "I" and "me," he is beginning to distinguish a few people around him by their voices. His face brightens when his brother or sister talks softly to him. He recognizes his mother's voice particularly, though he often seems less content with it. He may stop what he's doing, slowly turn toward her voice, mouth his fist, and frown, squirm, or fuss. His father may more readily produce a smile, as well as the most prolonged period of responsiveness. This difference may be based on an early association of cues, or a kind of discrimination. Father may well be more relaxed, the exchange with his baby more pure than mother's, who may be distracted by other children and her caretaking duties. By this time, all the cues of feeding, her voice, smells, and presence have heightened significance for the baby.

Adding it all up, the baby is getting ready for the surge of growth and development ahead.

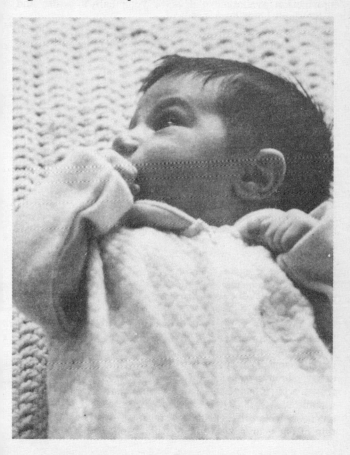

THE FIRST MONTH

Motor Development	Language
### Gross Motor	### Vocalizing
Virtually all arm, leg, and hand movements are still reflexive. On back, tonic neck reflex (fencer's position) still predominates. Thrusts arms and legs in play.	Besides crying, begins small throaty sounds.
	### Responding
Unsupported head sags, flops forward or back. On tummy, turns head to clear nose from bed; lifts head briefly.	Responds to voice.
Rolls partway to side from back.	
When angry, some babies can propel their bodies the full length of crib by digging their heels into mattress and thrusting out with their legs.	
### Sitting	
May hold head in line with back when pulled to sitting position.	
### Fine Motor	
Generally keeps hands fisted or slightly open. When fingers are pried open, grasps handle of rattle but drops it quickly.	
Stares at object; does not reach. Hands and feet will clasp an object if no closer than six to eight inches, not farther than 24 inches, and if object is moving slowly enough (one foot per second).	
Coordinates eyes more.	

Please do not regard this chart as a rigid timetable. Babies are unpredictable. Some perform an activity earlier or later than the chart indicates.

Mental	Social
### Sensory Response	### Personal
Prefers patterns to any kind of color, brightness, or size.	Responds positively to comfort and satisfaction; negatively to pain.
### Attention Span	Adjusts posture to body of person holding him. Grasps, clasps people. Roots and sucks at breast.
Alert about one out of every ten hours. Vague, indirect regard and expression most of waking hours.	### Interaction
### Eye-Hand Coordination	May recognize parent's voice. Most of the time expression is vague and impassive.
Coordinates eyes sideways and up and down in regarding light or object. Follows toy from side to center of his body. Becomes excited when he sees a person or a toy; regards them only if in his line of vision. "Loses" them if at center of eye too long.	May smile back at face or voice.
	Eyes fix on mother's face in response to her smile. Makes eye-to-eye contact. Regards faces and quiets down.
### Memory	### Cultural Self-Help/Routines
Remembers object that reappears within 2½ seconds. Expects feedings at a certain interval.	Daily patterns of sleeping, crying, and eating are highly disorganized. Two night feedings; five or six daily.
### Body and Object Awareness	
Quiets to holding and faces. Cries deliberately for assistance.	Moves bowels three or four times daily.

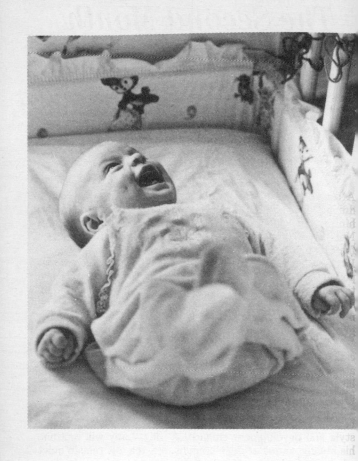

style, and let the moment surprise you. Do NOT stay within
his response repertoire in order to give it a proper polish
whenever you can. This will happen, but this is only automatic, and once you get it, don't worry, we're going to answer
through his development the stand of view. Look forward.
you'll be happy just to let his mannerisms style of the future
relax and let it grow whenever WA in bulk we praise and
smile.

The Second Month

THE SMILER

After your baby's busy adjustment to life in a new world during his first month, the relative calm of the second gives him a chance to grow dramatically and to socialize more. Not just a new plaything, he is becoming entrenched as a family member. He is also growing before your very eyes. In these next few months, some babies gain as much as two pounds a month. Your one-month-old is beginning to learn to control his head. It is steadier now and he holds it up occasionally at a 45-degree angle to look around for a few minutes. Voluntary grasping is already replacing his reflex grasp.

When he is calm, his movements are rarely jerky or staccato. But when he is upset or hungry, he reverts immediately to his earlier jumps and jerks. His chin quivers and his arms and legs tremble. A screaming child or a door slamming down the hall will make him startle, throw out his arms and legs, and arch his back. Even so, his movements become smoother every day and simple patterns of personal style and development surface. A quiet baby will continue his steady course of development, sleep a lot, remain quiet when awake, and probably eat well. An active baby may make you feel you are on a mad roller coaster as he careens through his developmental ups and downs. Most exciting, your baby is beginning to learn to adapt some of his inborn reflex abilities to new situations and to look at people and smile.

Routines and Regularity

By this time, your two-month-old may be quite regular in his demands. He may drink as much as thirty-five ounces of milk a day. He wants his daytime feedings (still as long as forty minutes each) at four-hour intervals and he is not one to let you forget them. His crying can become so insistent it resounds throughout the house and disturbs everyone.

The baby probably will be sleeping through the night feeding by now so that by the fifth week his nighttime sleep lasts as long as seven hours. This brings his regular daily feedings to five, with perhaps an occasional bottle once in a while at night or during the day. At seven weeks, he will sleep seven and a half to eight hours, until six or later in the morning. Usually babies will sleep through the night feeding when they are around eleven pounds in weight. Some gain this weight earlier and some later. Some two-month-olds, especially quiet ones, will still demand a feeding every four hours day or night because they do not tire enough to lengthen their night's sleep. For some, almost nothing will change this pattern except the baby himself.

During the day your baby will probably be wide awake for as many as ten hours now—taking one- to three-hour naps. An active baby's wiry movements may fill all ten of them. When put on his back, he fairly whirrs with activity, cycling his arms around his head, bicycling his legs, and twisting his body from side to side. He has a little trouble with more refined movements. If his cycling arms have to zero in on his mouth, he has to stab repeatedly to get his thumb into it.

Sometimes precocious physical activity can get the baby into trouble simply because you do not expect such prowess. His arching and flexing can turn him completely over onto his tummy or pull him off a table or bed. The mother of an active infant should start to check possible hazards as early as the second month. She also has to consider how to keep him covered at night. Since movement is an important outlet for an active baby, a sleeping bag is probably the best solution, because his arms are free and he can move unhampered. If he has to spend at least half his twenty-four hours in sleep, he should not be harnessed or tied down. His freedom is important to his happiness, his physical development, and maybe even his eventual view of the world.

Just as he begins to eat and sleep regularly, your baby will still cry at fairly predictable intervals every day. At the end of the day, he is likely to fuss on and off for about an hour. Some babies almost totally disintegrate at day's end. They may stiffen, cut down their activity, and seem to concentrate their energy in deep breaths ending in bursts of steady, high-pitched wails. Their color may change to purple and they may even seem to stop breathing, then quiet, yawn, and start crying again. (Infants before the second year will not actually stop breathing long enough to pass out.)

Nothing works to quiet this kind of baby. He will probably refuse to fit into any position offered and try wriggling out of your arms. Vigorous rocking or rapid walking with him in your arms may quiet him briefly, but as soon as these efforts stop, he will cry strenuously again. Research conducted under the direction of Dr. Lewis P. Lipsitt of Brown University by one of his associates, Dr. Leonore DeLucia, found that rocking a child when he cried only reinforced and encouraged greater periods of crying; whereas rocking him when he was quiet encouraged more quiet periods and less fussing.

Hunger is not the problem. You might be able to make him take an ounce or two of formula as he fusses, but he really is uninterested and usually spits it up as he becomes more and more active. He is more likely to eat at the end of his crying jag.

There is no magic way to interfere with this period. Babies this age cry a lot because they sense the frustrating imbalance between their sophisticated sensory apparatus and their almost total physical disability. Time and maturation will take care of this. Several days may pass without much fretting, followed by a third or fourth of nonstop sound, as if the baby were making up for lost time.

Actually the baby is beginning to compensate for his crying jags and that first month of fussing and disorganization. His smile, a thoroughly ingratiating response, has appeared,

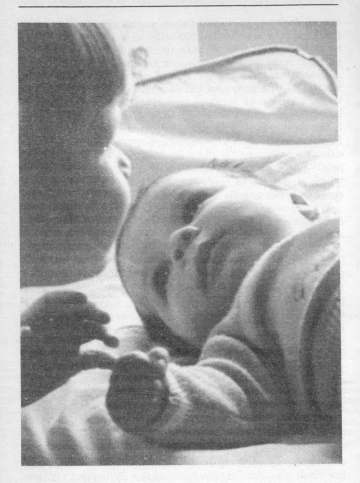

and other positive emotions counterbalance his expressions of discomfort or disgust. By two months, the expression of disgust is a full-fledged grimace to new bitter, sour, or salty tastes. Some infants even gag, choke, turn purple, frown, clench their jaws, and turn away. Now, however, the baby also responds to attention and seems to feel it is desirable enough to try to get. Most babies' responsive periods after feedings have lengthened, for some to as much as an hour and a half. After he has taken the first part of his feeding, he may pause to look around or to smile into your face. Although exasperating for a hurried mother, this play is wonderful to a baby. As Dr. Jacob L. Gewirtz of the National Institute of Health says, "The biologically satisfied infant is quite the opposite of the passive and unresponsive being he is pictured to be in the widely held theories of Freud. The highly responsive infant actively, regularly, and extensively interacts with his environment when his organic needs are satisfied. In fact he seems to seek stimulation which is ever more complex as he moves to each higher stage of development."

When people are around, the baby can gradually work up a slow smile and a bicycling performance. He performs his acrobatics most adroitly for an audience. When people are particularly sensitive to him, he can keep responding for as long as twenty minutes before he disintegrates with exhaustion. An active baby will arch, turn, twist, and kick so much that even you feel exhausted. Even when he is fussy, a brother or sister can amuse him. Alone, he has his own ways to quiet himself—sucking his fist or fingers, turning his head, looking at a fluttering curtain, or listening to the sounds of mother. Almost imperceptibly, his fussing slips into sociability, and usually by the end of the second month your baby is directing a lot of his energy elsewhere. For most parents, the beginning of this change is apparent only in retrospect. You may still tense expectantly for the evening fusses long after baby has turned them off himself.

Some babies begin showing preferences for one side of the body rather than the other or for a sleep position. The baby may suck his right first, look out of the crib's right side, and keep his head to the right in his infant chair. By the sixth week, the constant pressure may begin to flatten his skull. When your pediatrician determines that muscular or neurological problems, such as a shortened muscle or damaged nerves in the neck, are not the reasons for this preference, you might try the following: Turn the baby's crib so he has to look out to the left to see into the room and look at people, or hang toys in the crib slightly to the left so he must turn his head to look at them. Raising the mattress an inch or two on the right side so that gravity helps the baby turn his head to the left may also help. You need not worry about permanent head flattening because a baby's head rounds as it grows during his first year and a half. Pressure on the flat side will be alleviated as soon as he sits up.

If he is nursing, your baby may also prefer one breast, an fuss, cry, or turn away when put to the other. This favoritism may relate to an inborn preference for keeping his head to one or the other side or even to a position in the womb to which he became accustomed. If putting the baby on the unfavored side first does not correct his preference, try to nurse him lying down or hold him in a more vertical position.

Most infants strongly prefer a particular sleeping position, such as lying on the tummy. Some infants seek a corner or the top of their crib to press their head against before they settle down. Analysts have labeled this an attempt to return to the womb with the head engaged in the pelvis. If your baby does not fuss much or tell you in other ways, this preference may become apparent only when he will not nap unless he is turned on his favorite side.

Parents often try to change this urge for a sleep position because they have heard that one position is unsafe or another may hurt his legs or feet. Actually, satisfying the infant's natural preference for a comfortable sleep pattern is far better than tussling with the pros and cons of others

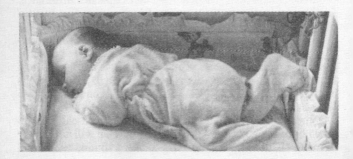

advocated in the baby literature. Infants, unless they are sick, will not choke on their backs. On their stomachs, they will not bury themselves in their bedclothes unless too many bedclothes are in the crib. (Heavy pajamas and sleeping bags in the winter preclude the need for many bedclothes.) Some pediatricians feel that orthopedic doctors overrate sleep positions as the cause of foot problems.

Early Learning

Your baby is beginning to associate and discriminate between many types of behavior. Placing him on his tummy may initiate screams of rage because it is the position he is put in for sleep, which he dislikes. If you put him on his back, he quiets immediately.

He associates certain people with particular behavior. He seems to have learned that if he screams a particular scream you appear. Before his meal, he sucks his fingers, but as soon as he is in your arms, his hands are of no interest and his sucking efforts are directed to the nipple. If you are breast-feeding him, he may refuse to take a bottle from you because he associates you with a different kind of feeding. It is not that he inherently dislikes cow's milk because his father can and does feed him from a bottle. But the association is so strong that his father can feed him only if you are out of the room and quiet. Even the sound of your voice in another room may make the baby refuse the bottle.

The baby concentrates his full powers to see, to pay attention to all kinds of cues, and to turn his head just to keep them in sight. Possibly size of the object makes a difference. In 1964, B. G. Bower, a scientist, indicated that two-month-olds do in fact distinguish object size.

Drs. Richard Held and Burton White of Harvard University also indicate that flexibility of visual response begins at about the middle of the second month. The eye's lens begins to adjust itself to the distance of an object. By four months of age, the lens of the eye comfortably accommodates objects at different distances.

Experimental data indicate that two-month-olds distinguish between sights and sounds. A newborn will not bother to move his head up and down to follow a sound, but he will try to do so for a gaudy bauble or a moving light. Two-month-olds also prefer people to objects and respond differently to them. Babies as they mature change their preferences from straight patterns, such as stripes, to curved configurations more like those of the human face. They grow still before turning their heads to a ball or a chime, while their response to people seems more immediate.

Your baby can recognize your voice now—even in a noisy, crowded room—but frowns and averts his head and eyes when a stranger talks to him. Although a sitter can try everything to quiet him, he may become fussy and inconsolable while you are gone. Though he probably cannot tell the difference between your face and hers yet, he can differentiate her handling of him from yours.

Even more exciting, he is beginning to acquire the idea of place. To see if three- to eight-week-old babies understood that a person's voice comes from where the person is, researchers at Radcliffe College used two stereo speakers that separated the sound of a voice from its source. The babies were seated before a glass partition separating them from their mothers just two feet away. As long as the speakers were balanced so that the mother's voice seemed to come directly from her, the infants remained content. But when the phase relationship between the speakers made the voice appear to come from a different spot, the babies cried, looked around, became agitated, and clearly indicated by their frustration that their expectations were being countered.

A baby also senses differences in his parents' proximity to him even when he is only half awake. For this reason most pediatricians and psychologists agree that the baby should not sleep in the same room as his parents. When he does, he cries out for them, requires more attention, and sleeps poorly.

Through visual and more active exploration, your baby becomes familiar with his surroundings and with particular objects, essential learning for all organisms. His perusal of the world in which he lives gives the context for all subsequent learned or instinctive behavior. Even if the baby can retain his newly acquired information only a short time, what he learns during sequences of quickly forgotten visual experiences may have a cumulative effect that lasts through hours of visual exploration. The accumulated knowledge then allows the baby to concentrate his attention on less familiar, unexplored parts of his world and so speeds the acquisition of information.

Even sucking, a reflex ability infants are born with, becomes a learning exercise for your baby. By two months, he sucks for food, pleasure, and learning. At this stage, fifteen to twenty minutes on each breast or twenty minutes on a bottle gives a baby as much sucking as he needs for nutrition. He can get at least half of that during the first five minutes, when his sucking is most vigorous. As early as three weeks, in infant begins sucking his own fingers for more than food. It is not because he does not have enough mothering. A baby with the best possible relationship with his mother returns to finger-sucking even after the most pleasant feedings because of the enjoyment it gives him. In fact, the happiest babies often suck the most. Some scientists have speculated that the baby is actually attempting to recreate the sensuous experience for himself and to compensate for the loss of his mother. As Dr. Brazelton points out: "When finger-sucking is invested with the memory of satisfying feeding, the contact with mother, and gratification of the need for sucking, it becomes very important to your baby."

Sucking quiets infants. It reduces hunger pangs and relieves muscle tension. Experiments have shown that the more active a baby is generally, the more vigorous his sucking, and the more it calms him. Although he may occasionally lose his comfort source in a startle response, the baby will try to get his hand back to his mouth so he can suck again. Sucking on thumbs or fingers rather than pacifiers has the advantage of satisfying the need for sucking independently of mother or the object itself. Pacifiers are not inherently "bad" replacements. However, the way in which mothers use them can be harmful. Some mothers overuse pacifiers to "keep the baby occupied" or to alleviate their half-conscious anxiety about the baby's self-sufficiency. Babies of such mothers can grow fat and passive by two years of age, happy only when their mouths are full. In these cases the use of pacifiers may reflect the mother's need for

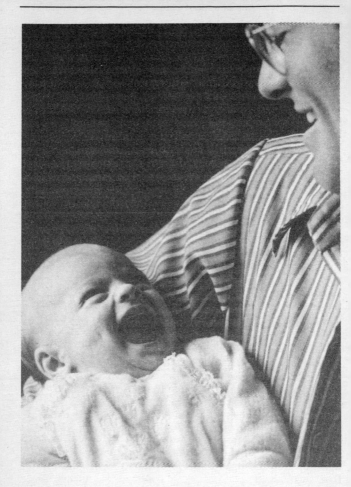

a "crutch." Although some mothers do feel a bit jealous of this first sign of "self-sufficiency," the very fact that your baby has learned a way to satisfy himself is a source of pride.

The mouth is also used for exploration. Sucking is not only pleasurable, it is one of the first "learning" experiences.

For the first weeks of life, your baby's mouth is one of his main channels of perception. In fact it is the universal all-purpose sense organ, although babies differ in their styles of using it. Some spit, others drool, some suck vigorously, others more passively.

Right from the start, infant sucking moves toward being fitted into many enterprises. The relationship between sucking and looking, for example, goes through three phases. At birth and for some days after, the infant sucks with eyes shut tight because he cannot handle more than one activity at a time. If the infant looks, tracks an object visually, or listens, he stops sucking. In fact, this disruption has been used as a measure of his attention. On the other hand, sucking reduces eye movements and so limits the baby's information intake. As sucking quiets him, he can focus more energy on one activity, like looking around a room and absorbing what he sees, and less on the random movements of his body. Unless an active baby can slow the rather frantic activity that absorbs his energies, he might not have time to add to his important visual development. The more practice a baby gets in doing one thing at a time, the better he may organize the neural patterns involved in a particular activity, and the better he can move to the next behavior he has to learn.

By nine weeks, or thirteen at the latest, the infant begins to such in bursts and looks during pauses. He may remain generally "aimed" toward the source of stimulation while sucking, but his eyes are not fixed or "locked" onto the object. Finally, often as early as two months and usually before four, the baby seems able to look and suck at once. Sucking's lessening preemption of other activities may belong to a general decrease in one-track behavior and a move toward the exciting and uniquely human ability to concentrate on more than one thing at a time. As Dr. Jerome S. Bruner comments, "Sucking not only serves inborn functions like nutrition, pain reduction, and exploration, it can also be diverted to intelligent instrumental activity that evolution could not possibly have preordained."

Research conducted at Harvard's Center for Cognitive Studies has shown that five- and six-week-old infants plainly work for visual clarity. While watching a lively color film of an Eskimo mother playing games with her baby in a snug igloo, infants changed their rate of sucking on a pacifier to bring the picture into focus on a lighted screen. The typical six-week-old learns first to "suck the picture into focus," but the moment it is in focus, his interested looking inhibits sucking, thus blurring the picture. The infant resolves his conflict between two good things by sucking without looking until the picture is in focus, then looking and sucking for a brief period. When he stops sucking and the picture blurs, he averts his gaze immediately. Gradually, the infant increases the time during which he can do two things at once—suck and look—and reduces the pauses between sucks to only four seconds. When conditions were reversed so that sucking blurred the picture, the babies learned to stop sucking on the pacifier and to lengthen the pauses between sucks to about eight seconds. Finally, the infant shifts from his usual sucking to a kind of mouthing that keeps the nipple less active. This reduced form of sucking allows him to satisfy his curiosity and to return to full sucking more efficiently than a full stop would. This "place-holding," as Dr. Bruner calls it, is a sequentially organized, adaptive strategy. It is the first signal of a mental skill that shows itself later in manual dexterity and language learning. Watch for it when your baby holds a toy with one hand and explores it with the other.

"Smiley"

For most parents, the most exciting second-month event is their baby's smile. If you look at or talk to a baby this age, he is very likely to activate his limbs and trunk and gurgle and coo until his whole body "smiles."

At this point, he is not really smiling at *you*. He is smiling at a human face. All over the world, real social smiling begins between two and eight weeks of life. Babies may even smile at human contact earlier. Some old-schoolers insist that first-month smiling is only a response to stomach upset. Some doctors say it signals tension discharge as the baby relaxes and falls asleep. But many have noted spontaneous smiles to human sounds or touches in the first twenty-four hours of life. One psychologist, Dr. Peter Wolff of M. I. T., suggests that smiles begin as barometers of mild surprise. Newborns smile to soft sounds during light sleep, but startle during deep sleep. A drowsy one-month-old will either smile or startle when a moving object suddenly appears before him. Perhaps mother's face appearing above her baby first draws a smile because of its surprise value.

Babies just naturally and instinctively smile at faces—pictured, sculpted, or real. Experiments show that infants under two months of age look longest at linear patterns rather than at curved patterns reminiscent of the human face. Presented with pictures of the human face, newborns do not prefer any particular arrangement of features. But from two to three months of age, babies prefer correct arrangement most consistently. (Remember that they can see much better, too.) They also suddenly develop a strong preference for three-dimensional heads rather than pictures or photographs of faces.

Babies smile most between two and five months because their smiling is still fairly independent of their social environment. Dr. Jacob L. Gewirtz of the National Institute of Mental Health established that two-month-olds stare at, grow active, vocalize, and quickly smile to unresponsive human faces. As early as 1946, Dr. Rene Spitz indicated that two- to six-month-olds are satisfied with any face. They will smile freely to a scowling face or to an ugly face mask with its tongue poking back and forth through the mouth slit.

Infants eventually learn that familiar faces are rewarding and unfamiliar ones are poor social risks. Smiling to faces of loved ones rather than to *any* face begins between seventeen to thirty weeks. As you bend over your baby, smiling, talking, and ministering to his needs, you encourage his responsiveness, and smiling becomes associated with pleasure and you. Cooing, smiling back at, picking up, and cuddling babies actually increases smiling. If this rewarding experience stops, infants gradually give up smiling.

An environment can encourage or discourage babies very early. In Israel, Dr. Gewirtz found that most one-month-olds living in nurseries on kibbutzim (collective farms) smiled readily to human faces. In comparison, only one out

A REAL CHARACTER

Smiling, crying, demanding attention—the baby is beginning to register as a personality. If you think about it, there are probably lots of things you can say about him. Here are just two infant personalities.

Baby A	Baby B
Has an intense drive toward motor performance.	Very quiet.
Eats with greed and gusto.	Relishes eating things he likes (at this stage, his mother's milk).
A gulper. He gulps down a bottle with the same vigor he shows in all other areas.	Eats efficiently, steadily, and neatly.
A light sleeper.	Sleeps a lot and deeply.
Wiry.	A little bit overweight (13 pounds) for his height but good-looking.
A "talker"—terribly interested in communicating with his loved ones.	Eyes are his best feature. They are remarkable for their ability to watch and track things and people alertly; even gives up his eating for this.
A ham and an actor.	Especially sensitive to people, does *not* like strangers, and fusses at sitters.
May be moody. If he becomes overwrought with his body English and gurgles, that charming smile changes with lightning swiftness to frustrated crying.	
Has a real temper.	Generally almost too good except for stubbornness.
Terribly disinterested in crutches. Fusses during the evening. May be fed formula, but shows the same lack of interest in it that he does in his pacifier and same emphatic response (spits it out).	Finicky and particular. *Very* discriminating about his tastes and quite assertively states some of his preferences. Strongly prefers one sleep position.

Baby A	**Baby B**
Commands attention with screams or charm—any kind will do.	Won't actively seek stimulation, but enjoys it if it is *his* style—gently, please.

Despite all this gusto, gains 1½ pounds and 1½ inches for a grand total of 11½ pounds and 23 inches.

of five of their institutionalized peers could. The kibbutz infants seemed to be in environments more conducive to learning to smile.

In another series of experiments set in the United States, Gewirtz and his team found that reinforcing infant smiles with nods, talk, and smiles, and discouraging crying, frowning, and fussing with expressionless faces made babies very "smiley" indeed.

All this adds up to a crucial point in your baby's life. He is really responding to the feelings and behaviors of others. This is when your value in encouraging or discouraging him clearly emerges.

Feelings are a two-way street—even with a two-month-old. Your baby clearly influences your behavior, too. Between one and one-half to six months, his smiling controls you. Your baby's laughter, crying, cooing, glances, and stares—and he uses a special variety just for you now—keep you comfortably near while he interacts with you. They encourage new responses from you, feelings you never thought you had.

Smiling and crying communicate important information about the baby's overall well-being, which, of course, greatly concerns you. A very young baby is a mystery even to his parents. You have to get to know him. His smiling and crying come close to your responses in similar contexts. They let you identify with your own parent or with yourself as a child. Crying may reflect all kinds of unknown problems that you might have to set right or it may even suggest blame or withdrawal of love. Besides, crying is a high-pitched, loud, lengthy, and very unpleasant kind of sound.

Smiling is easily interpreted as appreciation, recognition, and preference for you. It may also preview other interesting and charming events, like calling to or reaching for father. Because most mothers see infant smiles as rewarding, babies biologically predisposed to smile easily and often may elicit more approaches from mother than unsmiling infants, who unknowingly might hamper her involvement with them. But you know by now that your baby is an individual even in how much and when he chooses to smile. Even if he does not smile as much as Suzy next door, he needs and wants you all the same.

To avoid any confusion, we wish to reiterate that a baby is not one month old until the *end* of his first month of life. This applies to every month. For example, when a baby reaches day one of his second month, you do not look for what is anticipated in the second month growth chart until your baby is a full two months old, in other words, until he reaches the day before the beginning of his third month of life. Our growth charts present the average range of developmental achievements throughout the course of a given month.

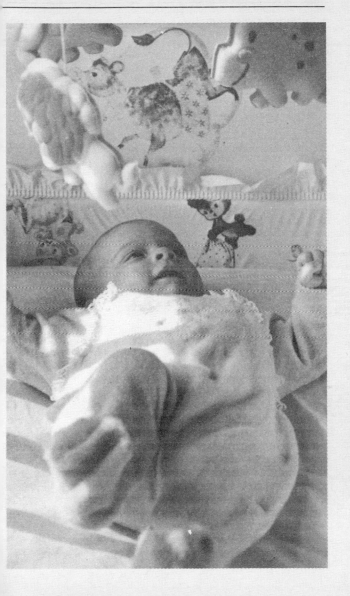

THE SECOND MONTH

Motor Development	Language

Gross Motor

Startles spontaneously (Moro reflex). Occasional twitches in hands and feet. Cycles arms and legs smoothly.

On tummy, keeps head in midposition. Can hold head up at 45-degree angle for a few minutes. When held parallel to ground at torso, tries to hold head up. On back turns head and holds up head recurrently at 45-degree angle.

Sitting

In supported sitting position, keeps head erect, but it still bobs.

Fine Motor

Grasps becoming voluntary.

Holds object for a few moments; may hold longer.

May swipe at objects.

Vocalizing

Small throaty sounds become cooing, vowel-like, but unlike mature human sounds.

Most vocalizing still crying. Interested in sounds.

Mental	Social
### Sensory Response	### Personal

Sensory Response

Startles at sounds or shows facial response.

Attention Span

Six-week-old not able to see small objects very well. Lack of focusing ability precludes three-dimensional vision.

Stares indefinitely at surroundings.

Eye-Hand Coordination

Coordinates eye movements in a circle in regarding light or object. Visually follows them from outer corner of eye past middle of body. Focuses eyes on objects at seven or eight inches. Stares at attractive, large, or moving object at several feet. Moving or contoured objects hold attention longer. Fixates on one of two objects shown. Reacts with generalized body movements and attempts to grab an attractive object. Retains object briefly as voluntary replaces reflex grasp.

After six weeks, occasionally glances at hand. "Hand regard" leads to deliberate reaching for objects. Objects that are placed in the hand are brought to the mouth for sucking.

Memory

Excites in anticipation of objects; begins to anticipate their movements.

Visually prefers people to objects. Stares at, quiets or face or voice.

Personal

Shows distress, excitement, delight. Can quiet self with sucking.

Regards person alertly and directly. Excites, orients, moves arms and legs; pants; vocalizes.

Visually follows moving person. Begins to prefer three- rather than two-dimensional representations of heads.

Quiets to holding, voice, or face.

Interaction

Most significant stimulation is still touch and oral, not social. Stays awake longer if people interact with him. May perform for people.

Smiles especially at mother, but also father and siblings.

Cultural Self-Help/Routines

May have only one night feeding.

Moves bowels twice, close to feedings.

Increase in wakefulness. Is awake as many as ten hours a day. Has two to four longer sleep periods. Sleeps as long as seven hours a night.

Enjoys bath.

(continued)

THE SECOND MONTH (cont.)

Motor Development	Language

Please do not regard this chart as a rigid timetable. Babies are unpredictable. Some perform an activity earlier or later than the chart indicates.

Mental	Social
### *Body and Object Awareness* Blinks at shadow of his hand. Begins to look at it as object for contemplation. May begin showing preference for right or left side. Repeats actions for their own sake. ### *Discriminating and Associating* Does one thing at a time. Clearly discriminates among a few voices, people, tastes, proximity, and object size. Associates people and behaviors; e.g., parent with meals, etc.	

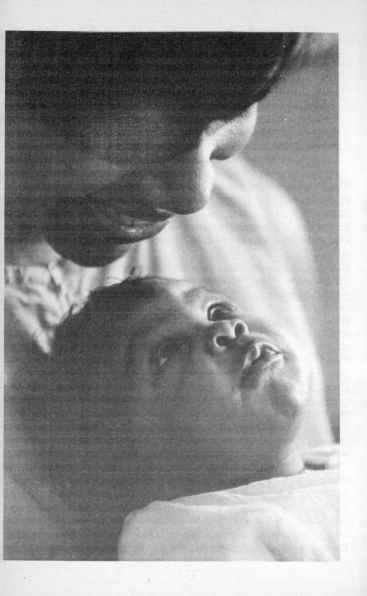

The Third Month

GETTING READY

The third month of a baby's life is generally easier and more rewarding than the first two—for him and his parents. Almost magically, crying nearly vanishes by the third-month birthday. The baby's increased capacity to engage the world with vocalizing, smiling, facial expressions, and looking at people, his better physical shape and control, and his new reaching ability replace his need to cry. He is an interesting and responsive personality. He can whimper in a special way when he is hungry, chortle as he actively responds to a human being, and squeal with frustration when someone he has been socializing with leaves him. Occasionally he may stop his activity, watch his mother or father, then try a slow gurgle at the back of his throat. Some babies use an expressive face. Your baby may widen his eyes, smack his lips, and grin broadly to a new taste treat. Placed in a position he dislikes, he may stare disgruntled at the guilty party. Since he likes to play and socialize, he smiles immediately and spontaneously with his whole face at someone he recognizes. He may search your face briefly, focus on your mouth and eyes, and become more active, kick his legs, wiggle, and reach with both arms.

Three-month-olds still respond with their whole bodies to many things and activities. Although they are still pretty much stuck in their lying-down world and trapped where parents put them, they are perceptibly gaining in specialized muscular control. Almost all babies this age can raise their heads while on their tummies and many can hold them up for long periods. This new ability allows them a new, bigger view of their world. Most can keep their bodies compact when picked up and hold up their heads with only a little bobbing when seated. They can sit propped in a lap or a reclining chair and even support themselves independently very briefly. Others when pulled to sit will still flop a little, like rag dolls. Some babies, in fact, can express their feelings very well with "body English." Yours may be able to resist persistent efforts to seat him by firmly arching his back and neck, or let his body sag to protest your interference in an activity such as looking or sucking fingers. He may also arch toward a desirable object with head, face, and open mouth.

All in all, the baby has become so delightful you are very thankful to have him. Your main hope is that you can match his new responsiveness with more of your own—a far cry from the way you felt just two months ago.

Night Owl

You and the baby have solved your first problem, too. His daily patterns of sleeping, eating, and being alert are clearly regulated. He sleeps better and more predictably. He naps quietly for two hours in the morning and an hour and a half in the afternoon. Although bedtime may still be difficult and some infants still sleep only six hours at a stretch, your baby is likely to sleep for ten and occasionally eleven hours by the end of the month.

Even though your baby may still cry with fatigue or suck his fingers as he turns from any new stimulation offered, he can help put himself to sleep with a definite pattern. His preference for his tummy or back is now essential. He wiggles, worms his way into the bedclothes, selects the fingers or things he will stick in his mouth, and sinks in. This nesting activity is often repeated during the night when the baby becomes half-conscious and must drop into deeper sleep again.

His patterns of deep and light sleep, called sleep cycles, are also becoming more predictable, as are his other routines. An active, noisy baby, for example, may be active and noisy even in sleep. Sixty minutes of deep sleep may be

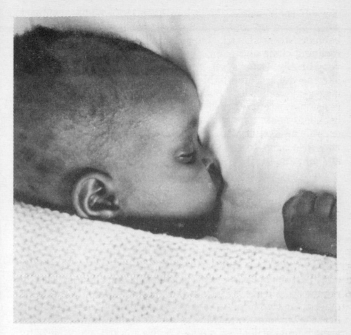

sandwiched between light, dreamy and more active states, semi-alert for a total of about three or four hours. Automatically and half-awake, the baby relives and reworks his latest developmental tasks.

He may suck his fingers, rock the crib, bang his head, move about, fuss, coo to himself, cry out, then nestle into his favorite sleep position and down again into deep sleep. These activities, which surface when the baby's state of consciousness allows, use energy left over from the day.

Nighttime might be one period when you can just drop everything and pick up your baby, especially if you have other children. But your response to his cries and activity will become a necessary part of his getting-myself-back-to-sleep pattern. With your encouragement, the baby may become a real live wire in the wee hours of the morning, dis-

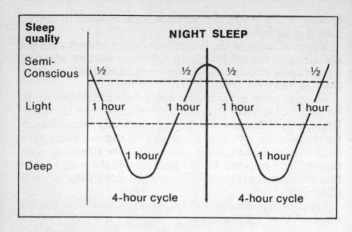

rupting the rest of the family and alienating you. Allow your baby to establish and use his own return-to-slumber ritual, even if this means occasionally letting him cry himself to sleep.

Infant Immunity

Babies need to undergo a program of shots and tests during their first twelve months of life that is as rigorous as that of any world traveler. Dr. Frank Falkner, professor of pediatrics at the University of Cincinnati College of Medicine, recommends an optimal immunization schedule for all babies. Unfortunately, many American babies do not get the immunization coverage they require because medical care in the United States is neither uniform nor extended to all Americans.

The average newborn arrives in this world already partially immunized by his mother. He has two kinds of natural immunity from his fetal stage: antibodies against certain diseases (diphtheria, for one) and/or allergic reactions to dust and pollen and the protein found in cow's milk. A natural way to encourage this inherent immunity is breast-feeding, which is why pediatricians urge mothers to breast-feed if at all possible.

However, some of the innate immunities against diseases and allergies are not long-lasting. Hence, doctors advocate a program of inoculations—often more painful to the parent than the baby.

An inoculation is basically a small dose of the disease to be protected against. Developing the disease from the inoculation is rare, because the amount is usually small enough for the baby's body to fight successfully and to manufacture antibodies against as if the "real thing" were attacking. Continuing the injections, as scheduled, builds the body's resistance to diseases that could kill if contracted naturally and all at once.

The American Academy of Pediatrics recommends the immunization schedule below:

Baby's Age	Immunization	Date Received
Birth	Hepatitis B*	
1–2 months	Hepatitis B	
2 months	DTP (diphtheria, tetanus, pertussis) Polio Haemophilus influenzae type b**	
4 months	DTP Polio Haemophilus	
6 months	DTP	
6–18 months	Hepatitis B	
12–15 months	Haemophilus	

*Hepatitis B is one of the nine childhood diseases your child needs to be vaccinated against.

**Haemophilus: a new vaccine against bacterial infections caused by the influenza bacteria haemophilus b; e.g., meningitis, pneumonia, and joint infections.

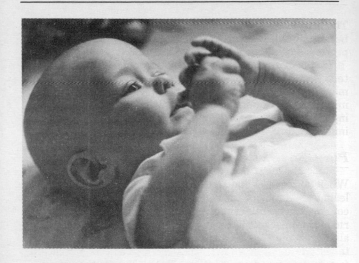

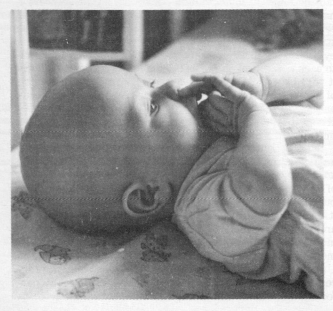

The schedule for immunizations may be subject to change because future research may alter the administration of present-day vaccines.

Your pediatrician can tell you about other vaccines to protect your baby against measles, mumps, and rubella (German measles). He or she can explain fully the need for immunization against diphtheria, tetanus, pertussis (whooping cough), polio, as well as Hepatitis B and Haemophilus influenzae b.

Play and Learning

When he is awake and alert after feedings, watch your baby learning and playing as he carefully explores facets of light, colors, shapes, patterns, sounds. He can play for longer periods now, up to three-quarters of an hour at a time. He already recognizes and attends to your sounds in the distance. He even stops his sucking to listen. He watches a face or follows the objects on his mobile as if they were a new experience each time. When your face appears, he calms quickly and he may concentrate on it intensely. As he stares, he seems to arch his head to reach for you with his eyes, and his mouth forms a circle. He shifts his attention to each new object on his mobile, and as it moves he follows it with his eyes. He can concentrate on a picture at the side of his crib or on a toy in the distance. At birth he can focus only on objects and people eight inches away from his eyes. His focal capacity extends with each month until by his third month he can see objects all over a room.

Some infants are acutely sensitive to the outside world and invest much more heavily in these watching, listening, and touching activities than in physical practice. This kind of baby may be slower to grasp an object placed in his hand, but more acute in sensing each new aspect of it as he turns it in different directions. He will stroke his cheek with it and bring it to his mouth for further exploration, while a more active baby would throw it out of his crib. Since large motor milestones are the most common measure in the United States for estimating a child's developmental progress, a baby like this may seem dull when he is really perfecting much more complicated skills.

One of the most important bits of early play that you will see involves something as simple as your baby looking at and playing with his hands. Hand-to-mouth organization, which begins as a reflex, is the first step in this process. As the baby brings his hand to his mouth, he begins to sense the gratifying stimulation at each end of this circuit. He brings a toy in his hand to his mouth, grasps things placed in his mouth, and so begins to appreciate the touch, feel, and taste of the things around him. Hand regard and play follow. The baby holds his hand before him and adds seeing to the circuit. One of the reasons he does this is that his eyes can work together now to focus on objects like his hands. Simply looking at his hands seems to prompt the

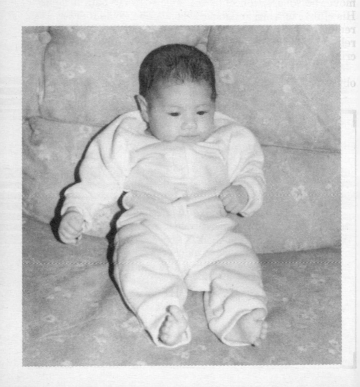

activity, and he plays with them for long periods. He watches his fingers move slowly, catching light, and at times intertwines his newly found toys. He looks back and forth between his hands, brings them together, giggles, and grins as they clutch each other. Then he pulls his arms apart and snaps his fingers away.

He seems pleased with combining the feelings of their motion and watching them as they move. He often explores his face with his hand, and as it reaches his mouth, still the ultimate goal of exploration, his fingers slide in and he begins to suck them. He circles his feet in front of his eyes for long periods, and in the same visual space his jingly mobile appears. The first time his whirling arms make it jingle and move, he sobers, concentrates, and gingerly bats it again. His efforts to whirl and move it become more deliberate. He remembers his behavior for he pursues his previous efforts religiously when he is wide awake and comfortable in his crib.

Your baby will also begin reaching out to each side for an object. If you hold a toy over him, his arms wave in circles

Some Suggested Playthings and Equipment

Birth to 3 Months: a colorful mobile, bright dangling objects, sturdy ring and dumbbell rattles, multicolored rubber or vinyl squeaking toys with safely embedded squeakers.

3 to 9 Months: a tot seat (for use in home or car), rubber blocks with securely embedded bells, hard rubber teething beads on rustproof metal chain, heavy plastic water ball with enclosed floating objects, smooth, colored clothespins, multicolored plastic discs, keys, balls, or rings on rustproof chains.

6 to 12 Months: high chair, playpen, spoon, cup, soft vinyl animals (and most of the above items).

9 to 12 Months: square or round block stacks, small ball, wrist bells, washable stuffed animals and huggable cloth dolls, heavy board or washable cloth books of familiar objects in bright colors, nesting blocks, small rocking chair.

at his sides at the sight of it. Gradually they come together to meet, grasp, and hold it. His grasp of the toy may still be automatic, but he holds onto it now voluntarily. Bit by bit, with practice, his grasp will become more systematic, more selective, and smoother. He may wave the object, although a baby less interested in physical activity will do this at around four months of age. Things a three-month-old sees become exercise material for his hands. He has learned that objects can be transformed by his own activity.

This kind of play has many dimensions. The baby's hand activity is self-instruction in depth perception, as well as in manipulating distance, appearance, and size. A three-month-old will move his arms more when a toy such as a shiny ball is close to him than when it is far away and unattainable.

The determined repetition that the baby shows in batting his mobile helps, too, in the growth of memory. The more an act is performed, the more likely it is to be remembered and a memory trace is established in the brain. The baby's memory from one day to the next makes daily relearning unnecessary. He can then add a new piece of behavior each time to his already learned repertoire of activities.

Continuity and Trust

He will reveal his developing memory in yet another way. He is learning to wait for an expected reward such as a feeding. Even if he cries about a slight delay, he may stop as soon as he hears your footsteps and lie in his crib expectantly as you prepare to feed him. When you pick him up to change him before the feeding, he looks serious and attentive but doesn't cry.

Since his new accomplishment is still fragile, your consistency in repeating the steps of the sequence is important. Even leaving him for a moment strapped to the changing table may "blow his cool." Unable to contain himself any longer, he wails with disappointment. Continuity of care, according to Dr. Anna Freud, is one of the three most important elements in a child's development, the others being affection and a stimulating environment. Young babies actually seem to enjoy repetition of an action or experience. At least in early infancy, a baby who is gratified much of the time and experiences a minimum of frustration can handle stress far better than a baby subjected to frequent tension or disruption of routine.

Loss of predictability in his environment, in the timing of patterns, and in styles of gratification can distress a very young baby as much as the loss of a loved one. In fact, unpredictability works against the very thing you may ultimately want for your child: sturdy self-sufficiency. Parents who sometimes encourage and sometimes fail to respond to their child's early dependency actually encourage his fragility. The need for some background of events one can count on is essential even to adults. If you are easily distracted from what you have led your baby to expect, his ability to build trust in his environment will suffer.

Obviously a perfect relationship in which a parent always comes through promptly with the "right" response is impossible. There will be times, too, when your baby cries just to let off tension and energy. But the degree of your consistency in answering your baby's signals is important. When a parent's responses to the baby's needs are usually prompt and appropriate, an important idea is sparked. The baby begins to believe and expect that his behavior, tiny as he is, influences his environment. How differently an infant must feel when no one responds to his wails—either because the parent is too busy with other children or because he is in an institution where dozens of babies are bidding for their parcels of attention. By the time someone does manage to come, his limited memory just does not allow him to recall that his cry brought about the attention. The belief in the value of one's own actions is vital later on. It is related to ongoing behavior, learning, and achievement.

Language Learning

The use of language sets human beings apart and enables them to impart information about things that may not be present and ideas that have no physical existence. Language is the most basic tool of communication that an infant masters. It develops in babies at widely varying rates and, therefore, at a range of ages. However, it does develop in a regular sequence. Although language learning is ongoing throughout childhood, the first two years of life comprise the optimum period for laying its foundation.

The language the baby learns is first the language he sees (gestures) and hears (speech) about him. In short, the infant's environment, his experiences in it, and his reaction to those experiences determine his language acquisition.

Language production begins with purposeful crying, then babbling, which is followed by repeating sounds and, finally, by the use of words and then groups of words. Until about three weeks of age, babies commonly possess a repertory of cries that express hunger, pain, and anger. By about four weeks of life, noncrying gurgly sounds usually appear. By six weeks, some phonetic syllables make their appearance amidst your baby's gurgles.

By two months in some babies and by three months in almost all of them, hearing spoken sounds becomes a definite stimulus to making their own sounds. When spoken to, a baby will look for the source of the sound, watch the face of the talking adult, change his activity (either by kicking excitedly or freezing to attention), and usually smile. As he smiles, he "talks back." Every part of the baby appears to go into this pleasurable social exchange, and every part of him shows dejection if the mother, father, or other caregiver ends it by turning away. Infants "talk" most when they are talked to. There is no substitute for the human voice for stimulating an infant's speech.

All the new social, physical, and eye/hand experiences of the three- to six-month-old tend increasingly to be accompanied by his own sounds. Just as the four- or five-month-old is seldom inactive when he is awake, so is he rarely silent.

Babbling, a major speech event, appears at about the end of the third month. At three to four months, most of a baby's babbling consists of open-vowel sounds. He says "ooh," "ah," "ae." These sounds, which are described as cooing, come before the infant adds consonants to his vowel sounds. The consonants *p*, *b*, and *m* are commonly the first ones added, as in "paa," "baa," and "maa."

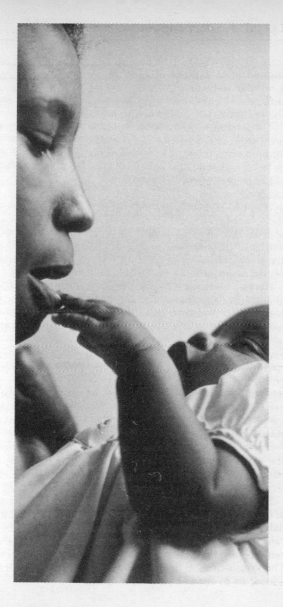

BABY TALK

Your baby probably has favorite sounds he repeats over and over again. He likes to listen to his own voice but will usually stop babbling if you start talking. Encourage your baby to babble by repeating the sounds he makes. Do not baby-talk when speaking to your baby. This makes his task of language learning twice as difficult, because he first has to learn baby talk and then "real" words. It is like mastering two foreign languages instead of one.

Discovering His Capacities

Your baby may be just beginning to associate a few of his actions with their results—a big step in learning. The hand-to-mouth organization already mentioned is one of the first examples of an activity style that still features total body commitment to an activity. As the baby brings his hand to his mouth, he begins to sense the gratifying stimulation at each end of this mouth-hand circuit just as he begins to realize that swiping at a toy dangling above him can make it move and jingle. He is beginning to learn cause-and-effect.

The baby's glimmering awareness that his hands and feet are extensions of *himself* is part of his awareness of himself and his difference from the world. He is learning about their extending, reaching capacities, just as he is learning his possibilities, limitations, and compensations for limitations. His whimpering for a change of pace when bouncing and vocalizing wear him out signals his understanding that he cannot handle a slow-down himself as well as he could with someone else's help. His waiting for you to give him back a toy that he has dropped means he is beginning to realize his limits in reproducing certain activities, as well as your role in helping him compensate for his inability.

Hand regard and play are also part of the baby's growing ability to reach out and grab things in his environment. It starts with the tonic neck reflex, which automatically raises the baby's arm on the same side to which his head and eyes are turned. Bringing his hand into direct view, which usually happens at around two months, is the first step toward the baby's visual control of his hands. Possibly his improved vision has something to do with this timing. He can blink at will, as well as automatically, and his ability to see things at different distances improves dramatically. One development enhances the other. When the baby differentiates his hands as objects for contemplation, his ability to pay attention for longer periods in his day jumps abruptly.

One-armed swiping at objects rapidly follows, usually with a closed fist. As the grasp reflex fades, the baby's fingers are freer to move, touch, and grasp one another. Eventually, the baby's hands will be able to meet over his chest or tummy. As the baby accumulates experience at fisted swiping, the movement will become more controlled, a slow approach of the hand to the object, sometimes accompanied by glances between hand and object and completed with a fumbling grasp. About the fifth month, the baby will be able to move his hand rapidly from outside his visual field to grasp an object directly and smoothly.

Internalizing Information

Despite the baby's efforts to swipe at objects and hold up his head, you may feel that he is far less active than he was during his first month. Remember that appearances are deceiving. Some fantastic things happen inside your baby at about this stage in his life.

In some research at the Educational Testing Service in Princeton, New Jersey, Dr. Michael Lewis found that three-month-olds have an image of the human face in mind. Three-month-olds at the Infant Laboratory differentiated pictures of normal and abnormal faces. The babies smiled more to a normal face than to a cyclops, though they stared at both the same amount of time. Dr. Lewis has also shown that babies older than three months have a short-term memory. Infants over two months of age become bored with repeated visual signals, but younger infants do not. A baby has to remember a signal to become bored with its repetition. This difference in memory suggests a major mental overhaul around three months of age.

Hanus Papousek, a noted Czechoslovakian psychologist, has noticed an abrupt increase in reaction and a "marked,

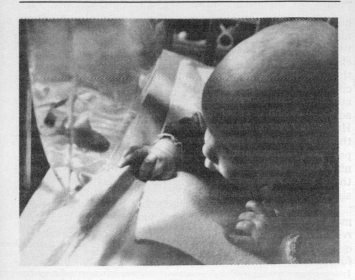

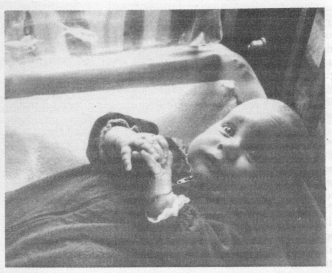

qualitative change in higher nervous function" at the beginning of the third month of life. He reports that in the first two months, infants followed from birth showed qualitative changes only in general body activity and vocalizing. From the eleventh week of life, however, they reacted more specifically and more appropriately to the experimental situation. Their vocal and facial reactions were like those of an adult, showing joy, indecision, uncertainty, and pleasure. Hand movements with toys, which were visually absent in the first six weeks, occurred in 30 percent of the observation periods from eight to ten weeks and then abruptly and significantly increased to 60 percent on the twelfth week. After the twelfth week, these movements again increased very slowly.

In your home, you can see signs of your baby's increasing mental competence if you look for them. By now, he may recognize you, other family members, even a few familiar objects. When he sees his bottle, he may brighten, arch forward, open his eyes and mouth, and wave both hands. In contrast to his smile for father, which he accompanies with more activity, he melts all over for you and smiles, crinkling his eyes and face. Your baby may also know what to do when he wants you to respond to him. You may see him search for you when you are reading or working in the same room. As he finds you, he coos until you return his glance, then fusses for you to come. When he wants you to pick him up from his chair, he arches forward as he looks at you. When you enter the nursery, he startles and whimpers for you to come to him.

Electronic machine print-outs of babies' brain waves support parents' observations and experimental reports. They show marked changes in activity and rhythms after three months of age. For the first time, baby's brain waves approximate those of an adult. The chemical balance and cell composition of the brain are also changed dramatically. Primitive reflexes disappear or begin to disappear at this time, signaling that a higher level of the brain is assuming control. During his first three months, most of a baby's behavior is beyond his control. His body simply responds automatically to certain kinds of stimulation. Now the tonic neck, swimming, walking, grasping, and swallowing reflexes start losing their hold on the baby's behavior. During the shift from reflex to willed muscular control, body areas governed by brain regions where transitions are occurring may be less active than before or after. Since neither the "higher" nor "lower" brain is working for the baby's benefit, the switchover means temporary disorganization. That is why a three-month-old baby will move his legs less than he did as a newborn. His quietness is only "momentary." Once a major reflex like the tonic neck reaction fades, arms and legs are free to move together instead of one-sidedly, and the baby will twist to one side and flip over less often. These signs alone should reassure you that your baby is getting ready for the serious job of engaging and moving about in his world.

The Importance of Stimulation

All this increased and more personalized responsiveness from your baby requires more sophisticated stimulation from mother and father. Since you are more confident, more familiar, and more attached to him by now, this should not be too hard. So much of what your baby has already accomplished has been activated or initiated by you—his parents. You are his providers, stimulators, shock absorbers, and teachers. You gratify his needs and adapt his environment for him—sometimes protecting him from it, sometimes organizing it differently, and occasionally exposing him more directly.

We have only recently begun to learn from psychologists, physicians, educators, and their colleagues how much the amount and kind of stimulation from the environment influences a child's development. Babies whose parents handle, play with, imitate, smile, and talk to them, who provide things for them to look at, listen to, and explore with their mouths and hands are advanced in attentiveness, visual pursuit, and coordinated movements, and tend to carry their early advantage over into later life.

Dr. Leon Yarrow, Chief of the Social and Behavioral Sciences Branch of the National Institute of Child Health and

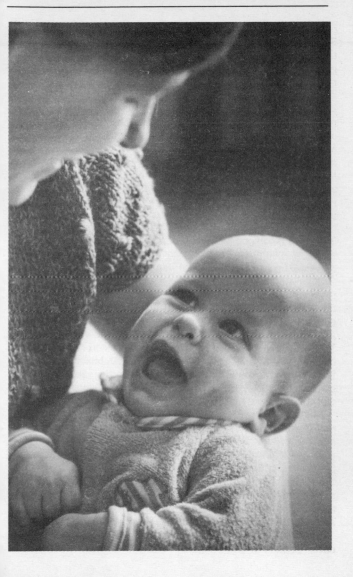

Human Development, says: "Perhaps the most striking finding is the extent to which developmental progress during the first six months appears to be influenced by maternal stimulation. The amount and quality of stimulation are highly related to I.Q. These data suggest that mothers who give much and intense stimulation and encouragement to practice developmental skills tend to be successful in producing infants who make rapid developmental progress." He adds that "appropriateness of the stimulation to the child's individual and developmental characteristics," as well as gratification of his needs and mother's affectionate exchange, also help mental development.

Like a shock absorber, the mother protects her child from too much stimulation from inside himself (like hunger or pain) or from the outside world (like cold or noise). She also enhances the positive aspects of her baby's world and directs his attention to them. Mother's sensitivity and capability in adapting the environment to her baby's characteristics actually boosts his ability to handle stress. Since he is completely dependent on you, he will need you to get him out of the binds he gets himself into and to help and protect him in periods of rage and frustration. If he propels himself to the top of his crib and wedges himself into a corner, come to the rescue and pull him to the center, even though you know he will just start all over and scream for help again. If you respond to his needs, you will enhance his and your pleasure with his learning and practice. Leaving him to his own devices may make him so fearful of situations he cannot escape from that he "turns off." You can also show him ways to extract himself from his frenzy and his predicament. After a few reruns, he will know how to turn around and get out of that corner.

If your baby is lucky, you will spend a lot of your day watching him perform and actively play with and enjoy him. When you comfort, cuddle, or rock him, he relaxes, quiets, and looks intently into your face. Not only is he stimulated visually, the whole tone of his body improves as he responds to your physical warmth and presence. A parent should try to see that the baby gets enough stimulation of his developing senses—enough sucking, looking, touching, listening—to give him practice so he can move to more complex behavior. The more stimulation he has a chance to get used to, the less easily he will be upset by new sights, sounds, and feelings. Infants are more sturdy and responsive than formerly believed. If you give yours enough to look at and to listen to, he will begin to be able to take much more.

Developing the important ability to pay attention does not just come with age. It depends on experience, too. Dr. Michael Lewis has shown that during a baby's first year of life, protectiveness, affection, approval, the amount parents smile, touch, and talk to their baby and, very important, the promptness and appropriateness of their response to the baby's crying and other signals all relate to his greater responsiveness. The more attentive the baby, the higher his mental capacity at three and a half years of age, as measured by the Stanford-Binet Tests of Intelligence. A baby who gets this stimulation also tends to be more responsive to his parent, less irritable, and more interested in exploring his environment and rehearsing his skills as they unfold in their developmental sequences. As the baby explores his environment, the number of activities that interest him increases. Dr. Jerome Bruner says: "The more a baby sees, the more he wants to see." He is building a vocabulary of sense experiences and forming abilities on which later learning depends: paying attention and developing specific, controlled sequences of actions. Practice in looking and touching things enables him to differentiate these activities from the rest of his behavior and then relate them to each other usefully until eventually he can reach out and take hold of something he sees. For the infant to learn from experience, he must have experience to learn from. Early perceptual experience prepares a baby for the later development of coordinated, visually directed behavior, which Dr. Robert L. Fantz says "is essential to active exploration and manipulation of the environment."

Lack of stimulation is devastating to the growing infant. His emotional growth needs encouragement and stimulation as much as his physiological growth needs proper food and rest. Saying that a crying baby "just wants attention"

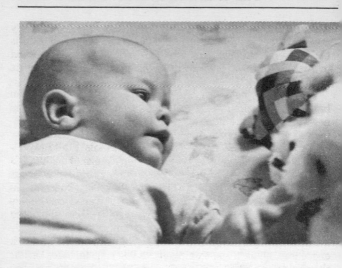

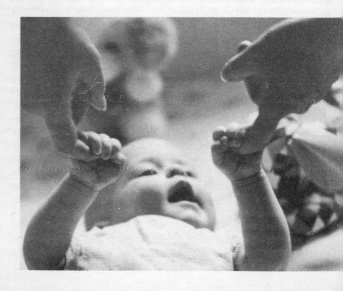

makes as much sense as saying "He just wants food." They are both real needs. Feed him if he is hungry, and if he is bored do not let him "cry it out." Try picking him up and bringing him into the family circle, where he can enjoy its richness.

Even if it is not always éxactly appropriate, a baby can handle and assimilate such stimulation. Referring to the need for providing infants with "a rich, varied, and appropriate sensory environment," Dr. Nahman H. Greenberg, research director of the University of Illinois' Child Development Clinic, says, "If, in his early weeks, the infant's environment fails to provide the conditions that bring about the fulfillment of sensory needs, the effect may be great. In later weeks or months, the infant with lowered thresholds and hypersensitization may react severely when subjected to the usual amounts and kinds of stimuli."

Since the baby spends a lot of time lying flat on his back or tummy, head to the side, hanging toys on the sides rather than over the crib is a good idea. An encounter with an "interesting" or novel sight can stimulate a baby to pay attention and can even keep a drowsy baby awake for as long as half an hour. No one suggests subjecting your baby to a ceaseless barrage of stimulation from which he cannot escape. Too much handling and anxious stimulation may create reactions like excessive crying, tension, irritability, even colic. A baby needs quiet times, too. Just as there is no one way to love a baby, there is no one way to stimulate him. The challenge and the pleasure lie in finding the ways and the amounts that are right for your baby and you. Sometimes the same stimulation can arouse or quiet a baby depending on his state of being. Babies differ in their styles of refusing stimulation. One baby may actively move to refuse objectionable stimulation while another's body may sag in protest until he feels like a sack of meal. They differ also in their ability to signal a need for stimulation. Babies who demand attention for themselves are easier to read. Overtures for attention and affection may not come from a quiet baby.

Babies are unalike in their sensitivity and responses to excitation and the degree of it they can stand. Infants who work hard at learning an activity may be somewhat insensitive and inflexible. You may find breaking into long play or practice sessions difficult. The baby fusses or protests until you allow him to continue. This determination reflects his serious investment in a task, which leaves him relatively insensitive to surrounding distraction. You can turn this quality into a learning asset. If you need to switch him to another activity, make the transition for him instead of frustrating him and yourself. Distract him, for example, with a toy. As you draw his interest from physical activity to watching the toy, he will be readier for another kind of play or for the necessities such as sleeping and feeding. The disadvantages of leaving the baby to his self-assigned learning tasks are that they limit him. He learns new activities from the novel stimulation you feed him.

Some babies need and enjoy gentler stimulation. A quiet baby's first surprise smile may excite you so much that you try to draw him out more. Instead of blossoming, he may become serious or turn away to look at an object or one of his hands. A gentler approach might be better. "Play with our baby whenever you want to" is obviously an inadequate guideline for this kind of sensitive infant. His delayed, slow responses to stimulation and his gentleness demand a special kind and limited range of stimulation. Outside this range, he may not respond.

Besides sensitivity, persistence may be needed to stimulate an inactive baby. Sometimes fears of making mistakes, "disturbing" or hurting him deter parents. Or a mother's overprotectiveness discourages a father's more active play. The muscular relaxation that often characterizes a quiet baby is an added deterrent. Yet leaving him in his crib or infant chair much of his day, undisturbed except by a smooth pattern of sleeping and eating, will only make a quiet baby quieter. You will help prevent his isolation if you continue to reach out to him.

Such a baby's even disposition, which remains unruffled by any of the usual events of an infant's day, may be the most difficult aspect for the mother, especially if she herself is expressive and energetic. Such a baby may not even mind his mother's forgetting to feed him at the appropriate time. This quiet, slow, or virtually nonexistent response to stimulation is known as poor "feedback." It is dramatic in babies with neurological defects, deafness, or blindness, but also occurs in physically and mentally normal babies, both boys and girls.

When a mother has to give so much of herself to a new baby, she instinctively expects a rewarding, cuddly dependence. Failure to get a rewarding response may make her avoid playing with her baby, question her and her baby's adequacy, or feel depressed and weary. This denial sets up a vicious circle—the mother's withdrawal and lack of stimulation further depress the infant, who responds even less and discourages his mother even more. A mother need not feel that she alone is responsible for difficult communication between her and her baby. The baby's sex and personality, to which he is predisposed before entry into this world, influence the exchange as much as the mother's personality. Mothers stimulate baby boys more than girls during the first few months of life, possibly because boys sleep less and cry more than girls. Yet research shows that mothers imitate and verbalize with their baby girls more than their boys. Many mothers do perfectly well with a certain kind of baby and less well with another. The same mother may handle a gentle baby girl with great warmth and sensitivity, while she may be utterly thwarted by a tense, driving, demanding baby boy.

To bridge the communication gap, look for things the baby especially likes. If he is quiet and contained, visual delights may be his "bag." Not every child has to be the all-American athlete. A fussy baby quiets when given things to look at or listen to. Unless he is very hungry, he usually will have longer quiet periods, and cry less if he is given toys in his crib, or held up and carried around so he can see what is going on. Once you do reach him, your baby will gather energy. You will find that the communication cycle will generate more and more reward for each of you in the exciting and definitely more active months ahead.

During the past three months, your baby has selectively explored his world through the only channels he has had—his senses of taste, touch, smell, sight, and sound. He has prepared himself for later explorations, manipulation, and control of the environment, and has established a base for another kind of contact with it, active physical participation.

THE THIRD MONTH

Motor Development	Language
Gross Motor	*Vocalizing*

Gross Motor

Switches from reflex to voluntary body control. Tonic neck reflex disappearing.

On back, keeps head in mid-position and posture symmetrical; lifts head. Moves arm and leg on one side of body in unison, then the other side, or arms together, legs together. Moves arms and turns head vigorously. When picked up, brings body up compactly. On tummy, holds chest up and head erect for about ten seconds; may lift head for many minutes.

Lies on tummy with hips low, legs flexed.

When pulled to stand, presses feet against surface and stands briefly.

When adult offers help with both hands, pulling-up reflex takes place. Walking reflex terminates. Can turn over from back to stomach.

Sitting

Sits supported. Can help maintain position. Minimum head bobbing.

At 3.8 months, sits with slight support.

Fine Motor

Keeps hands predominantly open; grasp reflex fading. May be unable to grasp object.

When shown a new reachable object, will bring both hands over lower chest and clasp them. Begins

Vocalizing

Cooing: one syllable, vowel-like sounds--"ooh," "ah," "ae." Whimpers, chortles, gurgles at back of throat, squeals, chuckles.

Cries less.

Vocalizes relatively independently of environment. Vocal-social response, e.g., to mother's smile and talk.

Responding

Listens to voices. Distinguishes speech sounds. Perceives syllable unit.

Mental	Social
### Sensory Response	### Personal
Hearing approaches that of adult.	Begins to sense that hands and feet are extensions of himself with limits and possibilities.
Discovers hands tactually and visually. Oriented predominantly toward things a yard away. Responds to mirror image if mirror is placed seven inches from eyes. By end of this period, can adjust the focus of eyes for objects at all distances. Visual capacities approaching maturity.	Smiles immediately and spontaneously. Crying decreases dramatically. Body tone and vocalizing increase. Chortles, squeals with frustration, whimpers with hunger, smacks lips. Visually recognizes mother. Begins to differentiate family members.
### Attention Span	
Attentive up to three-quarters of an hour at a time.	Strong interest in looking at human face.
### Eye-Hand Coordination	### Interaction
Follows an object with eyes and head from side to side of body for at least ten seconds as it is slowly moved about a couple of feet in front of face. Responds facially to object. Concentrates on picture or toy close up or in distance. Glances from one object to another. Regards dangling object at middle of body promptly.	Responds with total body to face he recognizes.
	When held, arms and legs push quietly. Orients and signals distinctively to each of several people. May stop or start crying according to who holds him. Cries differently when mother leaves versus other people. Smiles, vocalizes, orients differently to mother's presence or voice. Tries to attract her attention.
Swipes with closed fist or reaches with two hands for it. Glances at rattle in hand. Retains object in hand voluntarily.	Turns head to speaking or singing voices, familiar person's sounds, an approaching adult.
Distinguishes near and distant objects in space. Experiments with changes in proximity by drawing in and extending arm.	Social stimulation becomes more important. Vocalizes when talked to.
Begins to use hands to explore objects, moving them back and forth. Begins to use mouth as an exploring object. Gumming small objects is favorite activity.	Regular smiling to another person becomes a way of life.

(continued)

Motor Development	Language
to swipe, but may be far off target. Reaches for object with both arms, starting at sides and closing in front of body; often contacts object with closed fists.	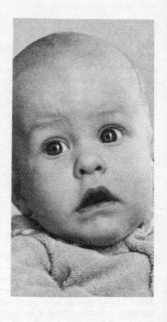

Please do not regard this chart as a rigid timetable. Babies are unpredictable. Some perform an activity earlier or later than the chart indicates.

Mental	Social
Gazes at hand and finger movements five to ten minutes at a time. Can create a single image of a nearby object. Alternates glance from object to hand.	### Cultural Self-Help/Routines Patterns of eating, alerting, and sleeping clearly regulated. One night feeding.

Mental

Gazes at hand and finger movements five to ten minutes at a time. Can create a single image of a nearby object.

Alternates glance from object to hand.

Memory

Begins to show memory. Waits for expected reward, such as a feeding. Becomes bored with repeated sounds or images.

Quickly calms to concentrate on a face. Attends more to three- than two-dimensional faces.

Body and Object Awareness

Watches hands and feet at length. Combines sensations of movement and looking. Explores face, eyes, mouth with hand. Begins to become aware of self.

Tries to prolong pleasing image or action by continuing to look, listen, or grasp. Repeats actions for their own sake. May associate action with result.

Discriminating and Associating

Stops sucking to listen. Looks and sucks at the same time.

Searches with eyes for a sound.

Responds to most kinds of stimulation and effort with total body. Switches over to control by "higher brain." Swallowing and grasping become voluntary. Begins to integrate voluntary and reflex behaviors.

Social

Cultural Self-Help/Routines

Patterns of eating, alerting, and sleeping clearly regulated. One night feeding.

Anticipates feeding by thrashing about or sucking vigorously at sight of bottle or preparation for breast-feeding.

Two naps, a couple of hours in morning and a couple in afternoon. Sleeps about ten hours a night.

Play and Playthings

Simple play with rattle.

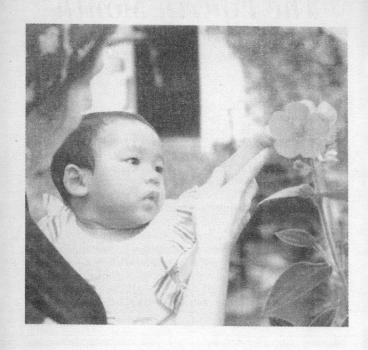

The Fourth Month

A VISIONARY

The fourth month is one of the easiest periods of life with
your baby, so enjoy it fully. He cannot get up, crawl about,
and get into trouble. He is lengthening his span of nighttime
sleep and staying awake for longer periods during the day.
He is responsive and cuddly, likes people, and smiles at
them. He has a repertoire of sounds that signify pleasure—
babbles, coos, chuckles, and gurgles. He will squeal with
delight and laugh aloud when you play with him.

Your baby is fun to be with—not only because of his good
looks, but also because of his responsiveness and obvious
delight in being held, bounced, cuddled, sat up, and
played with.

By four months of age, babies and their families shape
up. As you cuddle your baby now you will probably find his
body strong, firm, well padded but not fat—and it "stays
together." His elbows and knees are dimpled. His skin is
smooth, spotless, and minus its newborn "fur."

Drooling begins by about the fourth month and steadily
increases with teething. A lower front tooth may be coming
in, although it does not erupt until the sixth month in
most babies.

Typical Behavior

What is a day like in the life of a four-month-old? It is hard
to tell at what hours of the day your baby will wake and
sleep because he is in a transitional stage. However, he does

not show the wide fluctuations in waking time of the four-week-old. Your four-month-old's behaviors are more defined and separate now.

He wakes up hungry, but often will vocalize to himself for a while before his hunger becomes acute and he begins to fuss. He quiets when you come, but his patience is limited. If food is not forthcoming promptly, he will start to cry again.

Sleep is not as closely merged with eating as it was. It may be preceded or followed by a period of playful wakefulness. When he does sleep, it is a real nap and quite different from the diffuse somnolence of the newborn. It has been found that three naps in twenty-four hours are typical of this age, though there may be four. Naps occur in the early morning, late morning, afternoon, and occasionally in the evening.

The best-defined period of wakefulness occurs most often in the late afternoon or evening. After eating, your four-month-old may play by himself for as long as half an hour. Then he may feel the need for stimulation and attention and

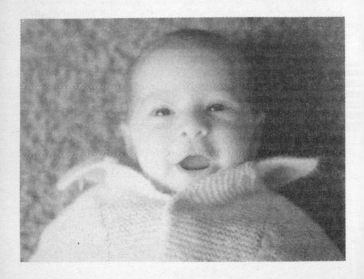

start to fuss. He enjoys a change of scene from his crib to a bed or sofa or a little walk in your arms. He likes sitting either propped up by pillows or in a baby seat so he can see and hear his world from new angles. Dangling toys intrigue him. He likes to be sung to and is content with mild and brief variations of experience.

Introducing Solid Foods

Feeding a baby solid food is something to which all new parents look forward. Why? Probably because this is a sign that their baby is developing normally and beginning to make the transition from infant feeding behavior (breast or bottle) to that of the child or adult (solid food). However, for the first four to six months of life, a baby receives all the basic nutrients and calories he needs from breast milk or formula. That is why pediatricians suggest that solid foods not be introduced earlier than the fourth month. There are many doctors who recommend that solid foods be delayed until the sixth month because younger babies are not developmentally ready for solid foods. Before that time, a baby's tongue projection and lip constriction patterns may interfere with normal swallowing mechanisms.

Another reason for delaying the introduction of solid foods is to allow your baby's digestive system to mature sufficiently to handle foods other than milk. Studies have shown that babies under four months of age are not able to digest complex foods; for example, cereals containing starch. The stool analyses of babies under twelve weeks have shown "largely" undigested particles of complex carbohydrates, fats, and proteins from solid foods."

Advocates of breast-feeding point out that by starting solids too early, milk will be crowded out of a baby's diet. Also, feeding the baby solids may cause the mother's milk supply to be reduced because the baby will be taking less at the breast.

An important reason for introducing solids slowly and carefully at four to six months is to prevent or diminish allergic reactions. The older a baby is when he receives a new food, the less apt he is to develop an allergy.

Your baby may give you some obvious clues when he is ready to start on solids. It makes sense for you to discuss this important step with your pediatrician or well-baby clinic personnel.

When we speak of solids as related to infant feeding, we are actually referring to semiliquid, mushy foods, including commercially prepared baby foods and table foods pureed in a blender, mashed, or put through a strainer. Of course, "real" solids require a full set of teeth.

It is important to add only one food at a time and to wait five or more days before adding a new food. It is helpful, too, to introduce a new solid food when your baby is hungriest. Of course, feeding a baby is much easier when the parent knows what to do.

The guidelines that follow may aid you in feeling comfortable about starting your baby on solids:

• Start each feeding with breast or bottle to satisfy your baby's hunger. You will be able to offer solids first after your baby has learned that these also satisfy hunger.

• When started, solid food should be given in a high chair or a baby seat rather than on the parent's lap. The restraining system should include waist and crotch belts or, if you prefer, a shoulder harness. Never leave your baby alone in the high chair or baby seat.

• Use a baby-size feeding spoon with a shallow bowl rather than a teaspoon. Holding the spoon to your baby's lips will enable him to suck off its contents. It will be helpful if you give your baby his own spoon while you are feeding him.

• Keep a box of tissues nearby to wipe food off baby, you, et cetera. It is a good idea to keep a piece of plastic or newspapers on the floor for easy cleanup.

• Generally the first solid food given is iron-fortified dry cereal. (Incidentally, parents should never give their children iron supplements without the advice of a doctor.) Choose a whole-grain cereal, such as rice, barley, or oatmeal. Do not give wheat cereal first, as this has a tendency to cause allergic reactions. Only one new food should be introduced at a time in order to make identifying allergic sensitivities easier. Use either home-cooked cereal that has been strained or one of the packaged baby cereals. Use no sugar or other sweeteners or salt in the cereal. (Any cereal can be sweetened with some sugarless, pureed fruit.) Put a teaspoon of cereal in a dish and mix it with breast milk or formula, adding only enough milk to make the cereal somewhat soupy. Give your baby just a tiny taste at first. If he seems interested (even though all you put in seems to come out on his chin), give him another taste. Scrape the cereal off your baby's chin and offer it again. Be patient. Swallowing is vastly different from sucking. It will be mastered as your baby matures. Gradually increase the cereal to one-third to one-half cup total, twice a day.

• Do not add cereal to your baby's bottle. To avoid a mess and save time, some parents put pureed solids into bottles with a big hole in the nipple, which allows the infant to suck it down. This is highly undesirable because the baby is neither learning how to swallow nor getting used to a spoon.

• Other foods that can serve as first foods include ripe mashed bananas, applesauce, and pureed potatoes or carrots. Strained cooked fruits (pears, peaches, prunes, apricots) and vegetables (string beans, spinach, beets) and meats, one at a time, can gradually be added to your baby's diet. Meats (beef, liver, veal) and chicken should be finely ground or scraped so they can be swallowed easily before your baby has any teeth. Either home-pureed or commercially prepared baby foods are good. Raw peas and raw or cooked corn kernels should be avoided because they can cause choking.

• If your baby seems disinterested or opposed to the idea of solids, simply wait and try again in a week or two. Never try to force your baby to eat. You can assume your baby has had enough when he turns his head away or shuts his mouth.

• Try to stay calm. Your baby will copy your attitude about eating.

• By six months, most infants take some milk from an unbreakable cup with handles and a weighted bottom.

• By six or seven months of age, fork-mashed or junior-texture fruits and vegetables will be enjoyed. This increase in texture should not be delayed beyond seven months. Ac-

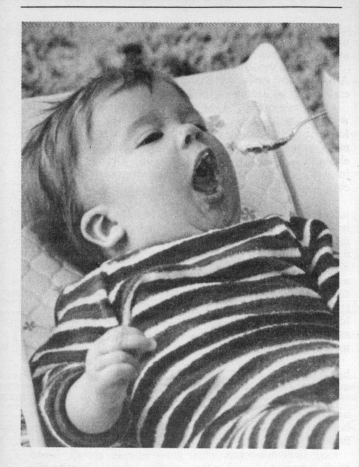

cording to Dr. Spock, when babies go much beyond a year eating only mushy foods, it is harder for them to make the change. Although when solids are first introduced babies sputter and make grimaces, this does not necessarily indicate a dislike for the food. This reaction probably is related to the novelty of the situation; the taste and the consistency are new.

• Between seven and nine months, minced foods, including meats, enriched breads, toast, potatoes, rice, macaroni, and crackers can be introduced.

• Teething usually begins between six and eight months. A bagel, hard toast, a teething biscuit, or a scraped whole carrot may be soothing.

• Between seven and ten months, babies can begin to sit with the family at mealtime and enjoy pieces of soft finger foods that can be gummed. High-protein foods such as minced, tender meats, cottage cheese, ricotta cheese, or chunks of soft cheese can be introduced. Orange and apple juice are also introduced one at a time, preferably from a cup.

• After a time, the breast-fed infant gradually reduces his intake of breast milk. The formula-fed baby may need help in doing this. If your baby is still taking a bottle, limit his intake to four 6-ounce bottles or three 8-ounce bottles per day. If he is drinking from a cup, three 8-ounce bottles per day are sufficient. Many parents find it helpful to offer milk at the end rather than the start of the meal. Babies seven to ten months old should be ready to eat three meals, plus suitable snacks, each day. From eating on demand, they will have moved to eating with the family. Between feedings, satisfy your baby's thirst and urge to suck with water, not milk or fruit juice.

• Do not introduce "mixed dinners" until each ingredient has been tried separately in order to easily identify and avoid foods that may disagree with your baby.

• By ten or twelve months, you can add some flounder, haddock, or halibut to your baby's diet. You can give your baby a bit of the fish you have baked or broiled for your family. Be sure there are no bones in the fish.

• By twelve months, whole-grain breads, cereal, bread sticks, crackers, hard cheese, egg yolk, pieces of fruits and vegetables, and whole milk will provide your child with a suitable, balanced diet. However, avoid pieces of frankfurter, popcorn, raisins, nuts, berries, grapes, and other foods that require chewing.

• Before the beginning of the second year of life, egg white, ice cream (because of egg white), chocolate, and honey are to be avoided.

• Always read the small print on the labels on all jars of commercially prepared baby foods to ascertain their precise contents.

• The Committee on Nutrition of the American Academy of Pediatrics has recommended that honey be avoided until a child is one year old because honey contains certain bacteria that an infant's digestive tract cannot deal with.

• All baby foods need to be stored in the refrigerator after opening and should be used no more than twenty-four hours thereafter.

Feeding Problems

When a baby begins eating semisolid foods, what should be a pleasant and satisfying experience for baby and parent sometimes is not. The usual time for eating problems to appear is when a child is about one year old. Variations in appetite usually surface then. The important thing is for you to be aware of some of the feeding difficulties that may arise, deal with them, and then proceed to make mealtimes as relaxing and enjoyable as possible. Healthy babies develop a good appetite early. Feeding problems may begin when parents worry too much about appetite and nutrition and try to force their babies to eat. Consult your pediatri-

---

Food Storage

REFRIGERATION	FREEZER
Expressed breast milk 1 day	Expressed breast milk 2 weeks
Open powdered formula 1–2 months	Liquid formula 1 month
Open liquid formula 2 days	Home-pureed fruit 1 month
Opened commercial baby food 2–3 days	Home pureed vegetables 1 month
Home-pureed baby food 2 days	Home pureed meats 2 months

cian about any change in your baby's digestion, or if you need professional advice in order to cope with a troublesome feeding behavior.

HICCUPING

One of the first feeding problems to occur is hiccuping. Pediatricians reassure parents that hiccups are set off by bubbles returning and are perfectly normal. They rarely bother the baby. Hiccups can be stopped by burping the baby and then putting him back to suck, or offering a bottle of tepid water.

GAGGING

When you first introduce a semisolid food to your baby's diet, you will find that as you spoon it into his mouth, most of it drools out. He may even gag from time to time. It appears that babies sometimes object to the pasty consistency of some solid foods by gagging. This can be overcome

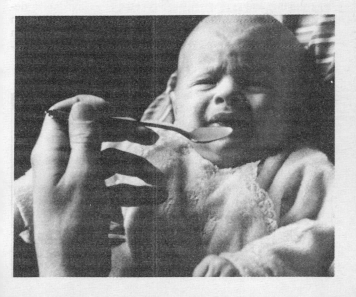

by diluting the food with a little milk or water and offering it more slowly.

SPITTING UP

Your baby may also resist the introduction of semisolid foods by spitting up. Try to determine if he is attempting to develop the skill of managing such food or if he simply does not like the taste. When in doubt, wait a week before offering him the food again. It is best to concentrate on the foods he seems to enjoy.

SNEEZING

There undoubtedly will come a time when your baby has a hearty sneeze accompanied by a mouthful of food. This is messy business. It is even messier when he proceeds to put his hands into his mouth, in his hair, and on you. It makes sense to bib your baby, and even more sense to generously apron yourself.

LACK OF APPETITE DURING ILLNESS

Usually in the case of an illness with fever, a baby will suffer a temporary loss of appetite. Infants should not be offered any new foods during an illness unless prescribed by a physician. Formula and juice may have to be diluted. Do not forget to offer plain water.

When your baby develops diarrhea, you should eliminate solid foods and fruit juices until you talk to your doctor. If your baby spurns the formula, dilute it by adding one-third water.

When your child vomits due to illness, let his stomach rest for at least an hour before gradually introducing tiny bits of chipped ice or small amounts of water.

After your baby recovers from an illness, do not force him to eat. The return of his normal appetite will let you know that he is ready.

FAILURE TO THRIVE

A steady weight gain is the most obvious indication that a baby is thriving. If your baby does not eat well or gain weight, consult your physician promptly. Of course, a decrease in appetite may be due to teething or simply a slowing down in his weight gaining, which normally occurs at about five or six months.

EATING SLOWLY

No matter how conscientiously you try to provide a pleasant mealtime experience, there are times when your baby eats so slowly that it becomes very exasperating. Try feeding your baby in a quiet room away from the distractions of everyday family life.

ANXIETY IN THE PARENT

Pediatricians warn that long before a child can speak, he can sense his parent's excessive anxiety and insistence at feeding time. Introducing foods in a leisurely manner can go a long way in preventing a row at mealtimes, and a variety of wholesome foods will be the child's main safeguard against dietary deficiencies. Being urged to eat, whether mildly or forcefully, can disturb a baby's willingness or even ability to accept food. It also paves the way to general resistance, a behavior problem to be avoided if at all possible.

Tune in to your baby's food requirements and responses. Above all, be flexible and sensible. When your baby stops sucking, he has had enough. When his mouth does not open for another spoonful, he is letting you know that he wants no more. Coaxing food intake is a mistaken kindness that annoys your baby.

Selecting Commercially Prepared Foods

While it is necessary that you feel secure about the quality of food you give your baby, do not let yourself become overly concerned. Infant cereals and baby foods are manufactured under controlled conditions to ensure safety, wholesomeness, and required nutritional values. Making sure that the manufacturers of prepared baby foods eliminate salt and sugar from their products merits the surveillance and support of every parent.

Cereals: Use instant, iron-enriched, dry baby cereals.

Fruits: Use plain baby fruits without sugar added. Avoid puddings, because they are high in calories and low in nutrition.

Vegetables: Use plain baby vegetables. Avoid those in cream or with added carbohydrates. Sugar and salt, usually added for the parents' taste buds, do not benefit babies.

Meats: Buy only plain baby meats. Mixed dinners provide very small amounts of meat.

There are a great many satisfactions to be derived from preparing your own baby foods, not the least of which is economic. In examining processed baby foods, parents should compared their cost in both money and convenience with other ways of feeding babies.

Making Your Own Baby Food

With a minimum of effort you can prepare safe, high-quality foods for your infant at an economical price.

SUPPLIES

There is on the market a very useful table-model food grinder. The food can be ground immediately after cooking and served at once, or the food can be ground raw and then cooked. This hand-sized grinder is handy for travel, too, since you can use it for preparing your baby's food at the table in restaurants or while visiting relatives or friends. It makes about a cupful at a time and can be purchased in department stores, some supermarkets, and health food stores. Plastic ice cube trays, the kind you pop out one at a time, simplify storage. A collection of small jars and plastic containers is convenient to have on hand. If you are also using commercial baby food, save the jars.

FRUITS

Most babies love fruit; others find it hard to digest. Some pediatricians recommend stewing all fruits (other than bananas) for young babies, but most feel that if raw fruit agrees with your baby, it is excellent. Canned or quick-frozen fruits can also be used, but they are usually packed in a sweet syrup that should be poured off before grinding or blending. (Strawberries usually are not given to babies).

YOGURT

Plain, unflavored yogurt to which you can add fruit is an excellent beginning food for babies. Yogurt promotes the growth of beneficial bacteria necessary for your baby's own production of vitamin B, a growth vitamin.

VEGETABLES

In preparing vegetables for your baby, cook or steam them until they are just tender, then use a blender or grinder. Avoid pouring away the water in which they are cooked. Use the liquid in the preparation of dishes needing liquid. You can use fresh or frozen vegetables, whatever the family is eating.

Potatoes, in addition to being a good source of starch, contain appreciable amounts of natural salts and some vitamin C. They can be baked or boiled and then mashed with milk or put into a blender or grinder. Boiled rice can be a good substitute for potatoes.

As mentioned earlier, as your baby grows, you can alter the consistency of the foods you prepare so they are coarser. You can start introducing grated carrots and apples. Thin carrot and celery sticks and apple pieces are good substitutes for teething biscuits, which are largely carbohydrates and sugar.

Child nutritionists suggest that since proper food intake is basic to every child's birthright, parents need to take the time to learn about the precise nutrition needs of their children as they grow from one stage to the next. All children develop food likes and dislikes based on what they are fed beginning in infancy.

Bon appétit to your baby and you!

New Moves

During this period, the family itself often shares moments of quiet and content, much to its collective amazement. Father is no longer listening with one ear cocked for the latest

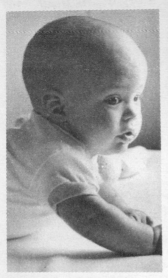
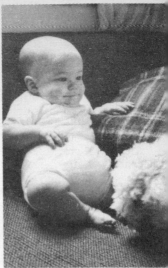

domestic catastrophe. You are beginning to feel rested and together again after a night's sleep or one of the baby's long naps. Baby's brothers and sisters, if he has them, have adjusted and are beginning to cope with their feelings about him. You can let toddlers fetch diapers, toys, baby food. Let them hold the baby briefly under your surveillance. School-aged youngsters can really help you to feed, bathe, and change the baby.

The baby is doing more things, too, and he has really begun to explore the outside world. He can reach for, grab, carry toward him, and let go of toys—and the whole routine automatically requires bringing the thing to his mouth for sampling. Through such activities he is establishing links between the realms of self and environment.

The more agile and varied use of his hands and his widening interest in things around him also contribute to more finger-sucking and exploration of his face and mouth. A study utilizing charts kept by mother-observers showed that extranutritional sucking occupied as much as four hours of a four-month-old's day.

The baby can be pulled to sit and holds his head steady when he gets there. Seated or lying on his tummy, he can turn his head and look in all directions. On his tummy, he can push up on straight arms and bring his head up to a 90-degree angle. He may arch his back, spread his arms and legs out stiffly like an airplane, and seesaw. He can roll over from his back to his side and sometimes all the way over to his tummy—which gives him new vistas to look at and automatically stretches his attention span.

After some practice, a precocious four-month-old may also be pulled to stand, maintaining his weight briefly. While only reflex stiffening, standing delights him and makes him aware of the act itself. If your baby is very active, he may enjoy standing so much that it stops his crying and makes him bypass a sitting position in favor of going all the way up. To get him to sit, you may actually have to bend him at the waist.

This is also the time to keep one hand *firmly* on your whirling dervish whenever you turn your back. Even if your baby is not the most rambunctious, he can slither from under a casually placed hand. He is much too active and interested in the world beyond to leave on any height. He can flip off a changing table quicker than you can move. He can work his way to the edge of a bed and drop off. If you have to leave him, strap him or put him on the floor, where he will be safer.

One by one, the baby will combine the motor achievements of supported sitting, arching his back, head-turning, and looking parallel to the surface on which he sits or lies to yield a marvelously new, three-dimensional space that he can make or change by himself.

Seeing is Believing

A four-month-old is fully able to delight visually in this new world. His eyesight is reaching adult standards. Unlike many infants in the animal kingdom, human infants are born able to see. Research has indicated that they can discriminate some colors at two weeks and they definitely respond to brightness values in the first month. A newborn prefers patterns to solids. His eyes and brain are developed enough to perceive form. He is aware of movement, probably the earliest, most basic perception. A baby glances at moving objects his very first day on earth and may follow a moving light within the first few hours.

But newborn vision *is* limited. Many things make up visual ability—the ability of the eye to see color, adjust itself to different distances, to see one image instead of double, to orient to moving objects, and to perceive depth. All these visual skills mature and start working together around the fourth month. The reasons are not yet fully understood. For example, how the brain and eye process color information, as well as the development of the baby's processing ability, still remain mysterious. Somehow by the fourth month, babies clearly see the world in technicolor. They discriminate the colors of the spectrum and even have preferences. They look longer at red and blue than gray, for example.

The eye can also see things farther away. In comparison to the seven-inch to eight-inch object distance a newborn handles, a two-month-old can follow a moving object *at least* several feet away. Studies on vision indicate that a two-month-old cannot follow a moving object at six or eight feet.

By the fourth month, the baby coordinates his eye and head rotations about as well as an adult who wants to follow an object with his eyes. The baby's head participates more and more strongly in tracking an object rotating around him, and he can orient himself toward the object of his attention. In addition, babies this age, like adults, use two different styles of head and eye rotation: When the *baby* chooses to direct his gaze to something, his head movements lead his eyes. When changes in the *object* compel his attention, the faster eye system leads the head. In either case, the eye and head move toward the middle of the body, probably because the eyes have to be centered to guide the baby's hands on either side of it.

Although scientists have not discovered as much about other senses as they have about these aspects of sight, available findings indicate that the baby also develops adequate hearing, taste, and smell around the same stage of life. What scientists really want to know, says Dr. Robert L.

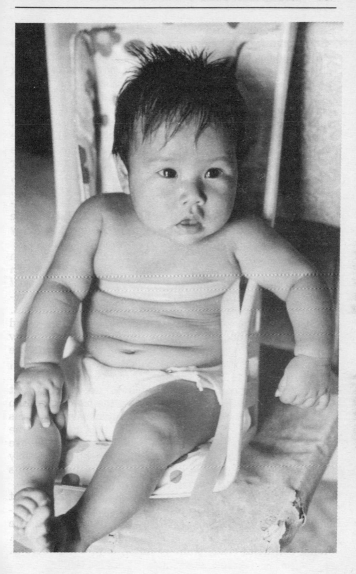

Fantz of Western Reserve University, is "when and under what circumstances the infant's visual experience yields useful knowledge of the environment." They already have a few answers for us. Your baby's ability to see his hands at different distances helps him reach accurately for things. Studies on baby animals show that a kitten's or a puppy's inability to watch its limbs as it uses them severely impairs physical development. In a now-famous experiment, Dr. Eleanor Gibson had six-and-one-half- to twelve-month-old babies crawl over a large sheet of strong glass supported by a wooden frame. A textured pattern was directly under one half of the glass. Under the other half, the same pattern appeared at a greater depth. Despite enticing toys and the entreaties of their mothers—both at the side that looked deeper—the babies steadfastly refused to cross the "deep" side, although they crawled readily over the shallow. Inde-

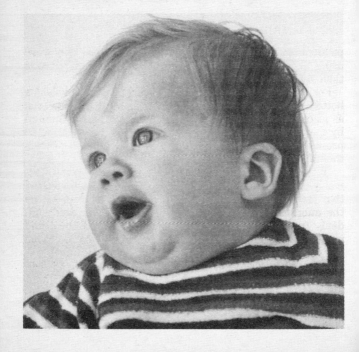

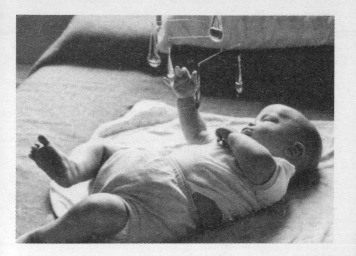

pendent of environmental reward or punishment, they were using their information about depth to what they felt was their own advantage.

For a long time Dr. Gibson's experiment established a bottom limit. Perception of depth develops at least as soon as locomotion is possible. But her experiment was limited by the infants' crawling competence. Babies had to crawl to prove that they could see differences in depth and process the information usefully.

In another ingenious experiment, Dr. Roger Webb, formerly of Harvard's Center for Cognitive Studies, indicated that *three*-month-olds see differences in depth and act on the information. When red and silver balls appeared suddenly from behind screens a foot away, the heartbeat and movements of seated three- and four-month-olds increased dramatically in preparation for grabbing the attainable— but not when the same ball was four feet away. *Distant* space may still be only a flat picture, a neutral zone. Without prior reaching experience, these infants plainly discriminated distance and started their visually guided reaching only to balls they knew they stood a chance of getting.

The First Tools

To describe a baby's growth, the old saying "One thing leads to another" should really read, "One thing leads to an explosion." The perfection of vision and the baby's ability to hold his head up allow appreciation of visual space. The evolution of increasingly efficient reaching also lets the baby appreciate and participate in his three-dimensional world.

You may notice that your baby can grab toys with either hand. This is partly because the baby has mastered the ability to grasp an object even if it touches his hand lightly or his eyes are averted. By the end of the fourth month, he can probably alternate hands to grab the toys or transfer a toy from one hand to the other. He may even wave it exuberantly, then transfer it and repeat the waving—shuttling it back and forth between hands like an amateur juggler. In imitating the behavior of one hand with the other, the baby may be becoming aware that he can do the same thing with each arm and that each hand is distinct from the other. This awareness is very important to his stockpiling of information about space. The baby also begins to see himself act when he repeatedly reaches for and grasps things. He starts to distinguish himself from the outer world.

If you would like another sign of this growth process, try one of Gesell's measures of mental growth, the behavior of a baby before a mirror. According to Gesell "norms," a baby will smile at his image at around twenty weeks of age. Hold your baby up to a mirror and watch him examine the faces there. He will probably attend most to his own image and perhaps smile at it. As his image returns the smile, he may become active and vocalize. He may also look back and forth between your image and you as if the duplication puzzles him. A baby who knows his mother's face cannot understand two of them. Calling softly to your baby as he looks at your confusing double complicates matters even further. His turning back to the real you shows that preference and clear discrimination are possible at four months.

An early attachment to one object—a toy or a stuffed animal—is another index of discrimination, as well as self-development, for the baby's interests are going beyond himself. Most babies do not prefer one toy this early, but some

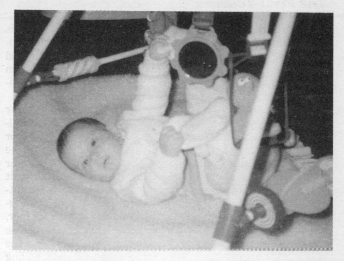

will. After exploring each toy in his crib, your baby may start reaching and playing with one special one, perhaps a set of clacking, plastic disks on a chain. In the months to come, the toy or anything else the baby identifies with himself by wearing or carrying may become a "pet." "Pets," or security blankets, as they are commonly called, can be anything from stuffed animals to shoes, a piece of clothing, a diaper, or a blanket that will be played with, cuddled—and dragged around when your baby is nine or ten months old. A "pet" will be slept with, chewed, hugged, loved, and "talked to." Removing it for brief periods, even for the best of reasons—like washing—may pose real problems. A baby can eventually identify so closely with his "pet" that a pediatrician can preview each step of an examination with it—put his stethoscope on it, flash his light at it, and thump its "back" to put the baby at ease.

The attachment of babies to such objects, obviously substitutes for mother, helps in the transition to independence from her. If you just think for a moment of how difficult this transition must be, you will realize the value of "security" toys for your baby. They give him another way to cope with

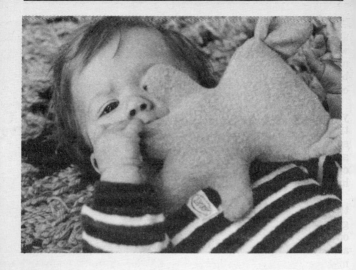

the necessary separations from you, as well as the other frustrations of just plain growing up. A highly active baby needs a soft toy for a special reason. Giving up action and play and comforting himself are difficult tasks for him. A friendly, familiar toy bear may just make him easier on himself. Rather than feeling threatened, a mother should be very flattered by her baby's extension of affection elsewhere. Only babies sure of their mother's love will stretch and grow beyond this critical relationship.

Play and Playthings

The four-month-old infant plays with his hands; later with his feet. His earliest playthings are parts of his body and those of his mother, father, or other consistent caregiver. Your baby's active involvement in play reveals the beginning of his budding social interaction with others, principally his parents. He also develops the skill to reach for and grab a toy, which he will mouth, bang, and explore with ever-increasing dexterity. Safe rattles and teethers are fine playthings at this time.

Toys that the baby can handle, move around, and change are good right now, as well as later on. Toys are to children what books and records are to many grown-ups. They are mentally stimulating. Toys not only keep a baby from being bored, they help him learn—about space relationships, color, texture, and countless other things.

For most four-month-olds everything is a game. Watch your baby as he finds he can produce sounds. He will practice them over and over. At each new one, he may stop in surprise and begin again. His face screws up and his arms and legs become active as his whole body works with the effort. As he becomes more intense, activity may break up his vocalizing for he still cannot carry on both at this pace.

Watch him as he is pulled to stand. He may actually chortle with self-satisfaction and pride. During his bath, he gurgles and laughs aloud, kicks up and down, throws his arms out and splashes water everywhere. He giggles with delight at loud screeching sounds he makes and squeals if his noise-making fetches you from the other room. When one of his sibs gets down in the playpen with him, he can double his playtime up to an hour or more.

He may even have a special game he plays with his family. As early as two months after the baby's birthdate, a parent may imitate the baby's cough. At first her cough and smile only attract the baby's attention, but eventually he coughs in return and starts an exchange. The cough, by the way, sounds like a smoker's dry hack. Later the baby initiates the game by coughing and smiling when mother least expects it. The game's value increases as the baby realizes his cough brings his parents rushing when he wants some excitement. While some coughing at four months may be caused by the increased salivation that goes with teething, the baby's "social cough," like an adult's, can be produced at will. Parents often credit the baby with inventing the game all by himself.

Recognizing authorship is less important than awareness that the coughing game, like most games he or his family will devise for him, is a real learning device. He learns that vocal sounds, like tongue clicks and coughs, are very effective in initiating socializing. He learns that his behavior can affect his environment positively—something very important for a baby to know. Above all, he learns how to imitate oral sounds, an ability essential in language learning.

By the fourth month even the most active baby will devote at least equal time to social contact. A familiar face can interrupt his most vigorous gymnastics. He will look at it, smile to it, and then try a compromise between talk and action. Picking him up prompts eager vocalizing, a real laugh, and looking at your face. Anything that disrupts his play causes displeasure. Since most early conditioning for play is on the back, turning him over onto his tummy may bring a roar of protest or make him dig his face into the bed and lie motionless until someone moves him. To condition your baby to like lying on his tummy, get down on his level and play with him. Gradually, he may begin to play on it, for a while anyway, just as a change of scene.

While most babies increase their responses when parents or sibs are around, some will do just the opposite. Your presence, for example, may actually silence instead of promote vocalizing. An extremely sensitive baby may interrupt his private sessions of cooing, vowel practice, tone play, and careful self-listening to cautiously watch your face and movements. Rest assured that in time he will cope with your appearance and respond to your sounds with his own.

More on Crying

By four months of age, having enjoyed social interaction with his parents, an infant may cry for attention. He finds smiling, waving of arms, and babbling to someone more fun and more exciting than being alone in a crib, playpen, or infant seat. Such containment devices are boring and frustrating to their occupants. Your baby will cry to let you know that he is lonely, wants attention, and is ready for play. Completely ignoring such cries may cause your infant to develop emotional problems.

You know by now that babies cry when they are hungry, uncomfortable, or tired and need to sleep. If your baby is tired, he may try to tell you so by wriggling in your arms while crying. Once laid down, with some gentle patting or

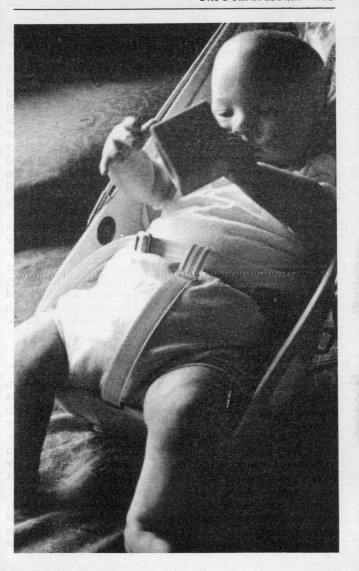

soft singing he will almost assuredly drift off to restful sleep.

Often infants will cry when they see their parents leaving them, even if it is to go into the next room. Your baby is used to having you near and feels threatened by your disappearance. He has learned to love you as you take care of him, and this should make you feel marvelous. If you have gone to another part of the house, occasionally call to and talk to your baby. Although he cannot see you, he is able to recognize your voice and will feel more secure knowing you are near.

Probably the most disturbing cry for a parent comes when it is time for the baby to sleep. His cry is one that could break your heart. When you appear, he quiets immediately, but the crying resumes the moment you turn to leave. This may happen when you put your baby to bed for a nap, for the night, or if he awakens in the middle of the night.

If you ignore the cry or let him cry it out, he will just become more lonely, and you will become more annoyed. Pat your baby, rock him, soothe him, and when he is calmed, leave! He will probably cry again, but after a few evenings, he will learn that he is able to go to sleep by himself.

A baby's cry of fear in the night is quite a different cry. It is possible that your baby may have had a bad dream, prompted perhaps by wall shadows, strange noises, or remembrances of things that occurred during the day. Whatever the cause, go to your baby, hold him in your arms, express your love, and then return him to his bed.

Exercising Your Baby

Exercising babies should be joyful play rather than sheer physical conditioning. Pediatrician Paul Dymnt, chairman of the Sports Medicine Committee of the American Academy of Pediatrics, has this to say: "The prevailing view seems to be that play/exercise classes for babies and their mothers are of no medical value, but if they increase the time spent between parent and child, then they can be of great psychological value."

Babies enjoy gentle bouncing, rocking, swinging, and tip-

A Few Suggested Exercises

You can do relaxing exercises with your baby for ten to fifteen minutes every day. An exercise can be done four or five times if you and your baby are having a good time together.

To relax his arms, put your baby on his back on the floor on top of a blanket. Holding him by his forearms, gently stretch his arms forward. Then lower them sideways, with his arms fully extended at his shoulder level.

To relax his legs, place your baby as above. Support his legs under his knees and move each leg gently up and down. Move one knee and then the other one up to his chest and then down.

To strengthen his chest and upper back, with your baby on his back, cover his hands with yours and cross his arms over his chest. Then slowly stretch them out to the sides.

To strengthen his abdomen and legs, put your baby on his back. Hold each lower leg and rotate gently as if he were bicycle-riding.

To strengthen his stomach muscles, put your baby on his back and cover his hands with your hands. Gradually pull him into a sitting position, and then gently lower him down.

A Jolly Jumper, which enables a baby four months and older to hop up and down, will strengthen his legs and is a lot of fun. It can be hung from the top of a door frame by a hook from which is suspended a thick piece of rubber that is connected to a chain. The bottom has a piece of canvas that wraps securely around a baby's middle.

Of course, parents can "exercise" their babies at home. Many go to commercial parent-baby exercise programs (offered at "Y's," schools, and other places) to get out of the house, meet other parents, and make friends, in addition to learning about how to stimulate their babies physically. A professor of pediatrics at the University of Southern California maintains that it is more important for a parent to cuddle and talk to his or her infant than to "fold his [the baby's] knees back and forth."

Check with the librarian at your local public library for the latest infant physical exercise book. You can also talk to your pediatrician about the pros and cons of physical stimulation for your baby.

In another section you will find a discussion of swimming lessons for babies under three years of age.

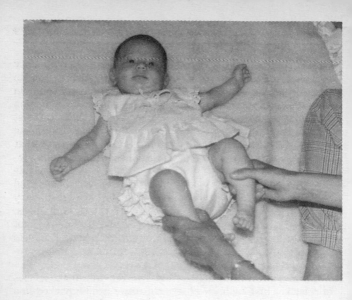

ping. Your baby's reaction should determine whether the movements are too fast or too vigorous. Signs that an exercise is enjoyable will include your baby's smiling, vocalizing, and a relaxed but active body. Startling, crying, frowning, or stiffening his body are warning signs of distress and excessive stimulation. Never use rapid, rough, or jerky movements. Of course, active or other play exercise needs to be avoided just before a baby's sleep times.

If your baby smiles and coos when you are engaged in playful physical activities together, you will know that you are doing them properly. If he frets or cries, stop immediately. After all, your baby is not tuning up for the Junior Olympics!

Visiting

The best time to take the baby out with you socially is during his first six months or so. It will not be this easy again for a long time. He is still eminently portable, light, and easy to carry. Soon he will be more aware of his surroundings and the people in it and may not sleep as well in an unfamiliar bed. Until then, not capitalizing on his mobility is a shame. In some ways, this is also the easiest time to take a baby along when you travel. He will sleep happily in any container you make him snug in. In addition, the motion and hum of cars, trains, and planes are soothing to most babies. A number of products are available today that make it easier to travel with a baby. Prepackaged formula that needs no refrigeration comes in disposable cans in ready-to-use or concentrated form. Also, there are disposable diapers, diaper liners, and bibs, as well as towels and washcloths saturated with cleansing lotion. Most baby preparations come in light, nonbreakable plastic containers. Unless you are going to out-of-the-way places, you need not stock up and carry a lot of equipment with you. Products like these are available at most drugstores and many grocery stores throughout our country.

Carriage rides, outings to shops, and excursions to houses of relatives and friends, where the baby can be parked in a bedroom, can help dilute sensitivity to strange people, animals, objects, and places and gradually expose and condition him to the world. Sometimes the baby is simply unused to coping with more than his usual two adults.

Baby Carriers

Take your baby with you when you shop for a front or back baby carrier in order to match one to his size. Make sure that the carrier is well made of rugged material because it must support your infant's back. The holes need to be small enough for his legs so he cannot slip through.

Also make certain that the aluminum frame of a backpack is properly padded to avoid painful bumps. Check the carrier now and again for rips in seams and fasteners. It is a good idea for you to bend at your knees when you need to pick up something, otherwise your baby may tip out of the carrier and you may hurt your back.

Inasmuch as a baby over five months old may become fidgety in a back carrier, remember always to fasten the restraining straps.

Traveling With Baby

Parents are a people on the go, and increasingly they are taking their babies and toddlers along on trips and visits. Families are traveling together by car, plane, train, or bus, and restaurants and motels are catering more to their needs. Although traveling and visiting with a baby present certain problems, advance planning and some simple precautions will enable parents to avoid difficulties and enjoy even the most ambitious outing.

A small baby usually travels well. If kept dry, fed regularly, given sufficient opportunity to sleep, and the usual warmth and attention from his parents, he will scarcely notice any change in his environment.

Your baby can manage quite nicely with less than his usual paraphernalia. A car bed will satisfy all his sleeping needs; an infant seat will keep him in touch with the world while you visit and provide for comfortable feeding; a sling or backpack will keep your baby as mobile as you are. Most motels and restaurants provide baby equipment, usually without charge. If you are visiting relatives or friends for an extended stay, most needed items can be borrowed or rented inexpensively.

If you are traveling by plane, try to secure a "bassinet" or bulkhead position. The number of these roomy seats is limited, so you should make such an arrangement as soon as you check in at the airline counter in the airport. For the car, a sturdy car seat is a must. A good idea is to arrange to stop for the night by 4 P.M. For other outings, a folding, umbrella-style stroller will accompany your backpack nicely.

With infants, the biggest problem is formula. If you are nursing your baby, accustom him to an occasional bottle in case your milk supply fluctuates during the trip. Let your doctor advise you. By far the easiest formulas to use while traveling are the fully prepared "nursettes." These are easily purchased and require no refrigeration or further sterilization. If your baby is not on such a formula, introduce it with your doctor's approval well in advance of your trip.

Other feeding methods are less expensive and less convenient, but will work nicely. Consider purchasing a nursing unit with disposable "bottle bags" to be used in conjunction with individual cans of fully prepared formula. Sterilized nipples and a can opener can be carried in separate plastic

bags. Bottles of formula may be made up by terminal sterilization only for the first twenty-four hours of your trip or
visit.

Diapers pose no problem. The disposable ones, with accompanying plastic garbage bags, are a real boon to the
traveler. Continue to use them if you are a houseguest.
It is a convenience for you and a courtesy to your host
and hostess.

For general cleanliness en route, tissues, lotion, a damp-
ened washcloth in a plastic bag, and moist towelettes are
helpful. There are prepared travel kits of baby products that
you might find handy. For your convenience, set aside a
tote bag for all your baby's needs.

At about eight months, a baby becomes more aware of
his surroundings and it may take more time to settle him
in an unfamiliar room. It is wise, therefore, to take along a
few of his favorite toys. Feeding should be no problem.
Prepared baby cereal mixes up into a nice meal at the table.
Baby food is available everywhere and can be eaten at
room temperature. Simply feed your baby from the jar and
throw away any leftovers. Bring enough of the foods your
baby enjoys and digests easily. Teething biscuits, toast,
crackers, and other familiar table foods will keep baby content while you eat.

If you have traveled and visited often with your baby,
bedtime should present no problem, but if this is a first
outing, be prepared for possible upset. By all means bring
with you any security item your baby prefers above all his
other playthings. Be hesitant to leave a stranger in the role
of baby-sitter in a strange house, at least for the first few
nights.

However, because of the excitement of new stimulation
and audiences, he may react rather dramatically after a
visit—especially a long one. He may refuse his food, wake
periodically throughout the night, and respond to your attention only to cry himself back to sleep after you have left.
His upset can last for several hellish days of crying and
whimpering at night and during the day. If hysteria does
erupt, a firm, consistent reaction is probably necessary.
Your distress is very likely to compound the baby's. A day
or so of calculated indifference to his turmoil and bids for

attention should help the baby settle back into his normal pattern.

If you do go out and leave the baby home, be sure the relative, friend, or baby-sitter you leave him with can be trusted to do things for the baby the way you do. Have her visit first while you take care of him so she has a chance to see the way you hold, handle, play with, and talk to him.

Most four-month-old babies know their mothers, and although about half of them will adjust when a stranger is near them, the other half will rebel. After all, no other person besides you has given so many different and potent kinds of stimulation. If the baby sees you and your friend or sitter at the same time, it is easier for him to establish a connection and to make the transition from friend or sitter to you. (Imagine how panic-stricken and abandoned you

Baby-Sitters

In *The Father's Book,* Ted Klein sets forth commonsense rules for baby-sitters that parents should also know:

• In case of illness or an accident, call the parents. If they cannot be reached, call the family doctor. As a last resort, call the police.

• In case of smoke or fire, get the child out of the house immediately without first dressing him. Do not call the fire department. Instead, go to a neighbor's house and then phone for help.

• Never open the door to strangers.

• Never leave a child alone, not even for a second.

• If the child cries uncontrollably, call the parents.

• Do not go to sleep, shut a door to hear the TV, or entertain friends while baby-sitting.

Occasionally when a baby awakes at night and cries out he expects to see a parent's face. When that of a stranger appears instead, the baby is disturbed. To prevent such situations, it is best for the parent to introduce the baby to the baby-sitter in advance. That way the baby will not consider the person a stranger and will more nearly be able to accept comforting from his temporary caregiver.

would feel if you woke up suddenly in the night to find everybody you loved gone and a stranger standing by your bed.) A little later, in the ninth month, all this changes even more dramatically, so you might as well take these precautions and use this stage of your baby's life to get out once in a while.

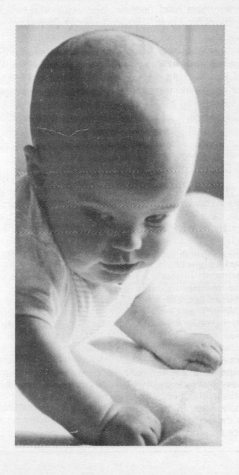

THE FOURTH MONTH

Motor Development	Language

Gross Motor

Moro reflex begins to vanish. On back, keeps head in mid-position.

Turns head in all directions, seated or lying. Holds head steady and erect for short time. On tummy, lifts head 90 degrees from surface, or on straight arms, or with weight on forearms. On back, may crane neck forward to see hands catch feet.

Lies on tummy, legs extended. May deliberately flex muscles from waist down, raising hips. On tummy, may rock like an airplane, limbs extended and back arched. On tummy, rolls from side to side. May roll from stomach or side to back.

If pulled to stand, extends legs and keeps body in same plane from shoulders to feet.

Legs have attained a degree of muscular strength. Can support own weight if held upright with feet against a flat surface.

Reaches with the arms. Continuously practices gross-motor skills as each one appears and matures: torso control, turning over, head control.

Sitting

Sits supported ten to fifteen minutes, head erect and steady, back firm.

Vocalizing

Cooing becomes pitch modulated. Sustains it for fifteen to twenty minutes. Begins babbling; strings of syllablelike vocalizing.

Voice quality normalizing; strong, steady cry.

Vocalizes moods of pleasure up to thirty minutes—chortles, squeals, gurgles, giggles, grins, laughs aloud.

Imitates several tones.

Responding

When talked to, smiles, squeals, coos.

Begins to react to a tickle. Remarkably accurate in turning ear and body to the source of a sound. By four to five months, can identify mother's voice from others.

Mental	Social
### Sensory Response	### Personal

Sensory Response

Vision approximates that of adults. Sees in color. Lens of eye adjusts to objects at varying distances.

Attention Span

May increase responsive periods to an hour or more at a time. Sustains interest in details.

Can play alone for longer periods.

Eye-Hand Coordination

Head and eyes turn in coordination and parallel to surface on which he lies or sits; follows dangling or moving object, sound source. Regards ring or rattle immediately.

Activates arms and trunk, looks from hand to nearby object, reaches for, grabs, and lets go of it with either hand. Pulls dangling object toward him. Carries object to mouth. Swipes with one arm and open hand but often misses.

Aware of differences in depth and distance.

Stares at place from which object drops.

Memory

Has memory span of five to seven seconds.

Smiles and vocalizes more to an actual face than to an image. Discriminates faces from patterns, people from things. Discriminates among faces. Knows mother. May resesnt strangers.

Personal

Vocalizes moods, enjoyment, indecision, and protest. Laughs while socializing; wails if play is disrupted. Shows anticipation; excites, breathes heavily.

Interested in and may smile at his mirror image. Many discriminate mother's image from his.

May wait for a feeding. Attempts to soothe self. Quieted by music. Clasps fingers and hands in play.

Interaction

Vocalizes to initiate socializing—coughs or clicks tongue. Responds to and enjoys handling; vocalizes when pulled to sit; not content to lie down.

Develops ways of getting and holding attention of another person.

Spontaneous social smile.

Cultural Self-Help/Routines

Interest in feeding decreases due to social interest. Recognizes bottle and purses mouth for food. May be ready for solids.

Predictable interval between feeding and bowel movements.

Splashes in bath, kicks, and lifts head.

(continued)

Motor Development	Language
Uses hands more agilely and with more variety. Mutually fingers hands. Unskilled mitten grasp, palm and fingers appose thumb. May take small objects between index and second fingers.	
Retains doll-size objects. Swiping still inaccurate. May look from object to hand to object, often misses but can grab it. Hands may meet below, beyond, or in front of object.	
Clasps finger and hands in play.	

Please do not regard this chart as a rigid timetable. Babies are unpredictable. Some perform an activity earlier or later than the chart indicates.

Mental	Social
### Body and Object Awareness	### Play and Playthings
Fingers hands in mutual play. Becomes aware of their distinctness. May smile and vocalize at mirror image. Begins to adjust responses to people. Becomes aware of distinctness of his act from external result; himself from outer world and other objects.	Shows interest in playthings; may prefer one toy (which shows awareness of something outside of self). Enjoys play, games, socializing. Doubles playtime if it involves socializing.
### Discriminating and Associating	
Aware of strange situation. Associates growing number of behaviors. Discriminates; may prefer one toy to others. May transfer a toy from one hand to the other.	

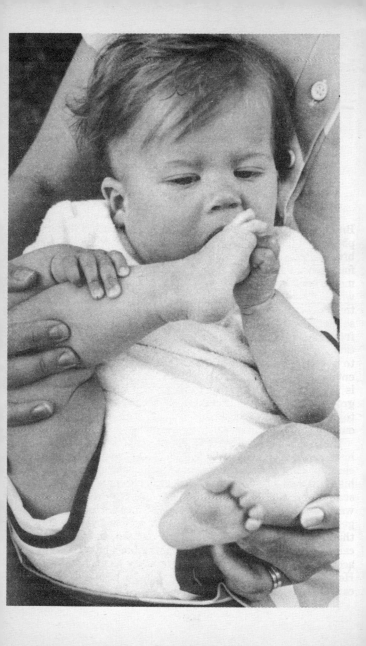

The Fifth Month

REACHING OUT

Brace yourself. For most babies, the fifth month is the first phase of a fantastic speedup of activity that will leave you breathless by the end of his first year. The quiet of the first four months is over. The baby's attention span, and that means playtime, has stretched to one and a half or two hours with a little help from you. True, the baby can still do quiet things, particularly when they involve differentiating himself from his world. He can turn now when you call his name from another room or he hears it in a stream of conversation. Mirrors still please him and he will even stop crying to look and smile at himself. This self-interest is very different from an adult's egocentrism. The baby's self-exploration is a healthy first step in extending beyond himself as he grows. His alternate mouthing of fingers or thumbs and toys is a way of comparing himself with objects in the outer world.

Because of his increasing ability to control the muscles in his trunk and lower back, the baby can sit propped in a chair for long periods. His increasing balance and control of his head and his new ability to grasp things while he is seated are very exciting. He is no longer content just to watch things or people that are out of reach. His eyes, fingers, and mouth work together as he learns and he wants things close enough to feel, hold, turn, shake, and taste. You can easily arouse the force behind this inborn integration by accidentally leaving your baby with a toy he cannot reach. He may suddenly howl in frustration as he discovers he cannot examine it fully.

The ability to reach and grasp, generally apparent around the beginning of the fifth month, has had a long, impressive history. In fact, the period from one and a half to five months is enormously important for early perceptual and physical development. First of all, the baby must be able to see before he can reach. He is born with the first necessary skill: being able to follow a changing or moving light or any small object that contrasts with its background. This visual tracking happens only if the object is on the edge of the baby's visual field. Once he is looking directly at it, the pattern it presents to the baby's eyes determines whether or not he will continue staring. In 1961, Dr. Robert L. Fantz showed that a newborn will fixate on patterns with clearly defined edges and high contrast areas—for example, bright, white stripes on flat black. This peripheral tracking and pattern fixation quickly develop into the central tracking and eye control that will enable your baby to follow moving patterns at which he is looking and to explore his world visually.

Around the middle of the second month of life, the baby's visual activity and growth surge dramatically. He learns to blink at an approaching object. His eyes work together so that they see one object instead of two. The lens of his eye is able to thicken or thin, depending on the distance of an object, allowing him to see objects clearly by the time he is about three and a half months old. This new eye ability allows the baby to bring his hands into focus, thus linking sight and touch by a double-feedback system. The eyes see the hand and what it feels, the hands feel what the eye sees. The eye control of the hand leads to hand play such as mutual fingering, then one-armed swiping with a closed fist, then jerky open-handed reaching in which the baby's hand often misses its target. Gradually the baby's aim improves as he looks between hand and object and his "direct hits" increase. Then, shortly before five months, the baby can bring his hand rapidly from outside his field of vision to an object he is looking at and grasp it smoothly. As you may have noticed in your baby, the progression of muscle control has been from eyes, head, and arms to hands, and from center to the outside edges of vision.

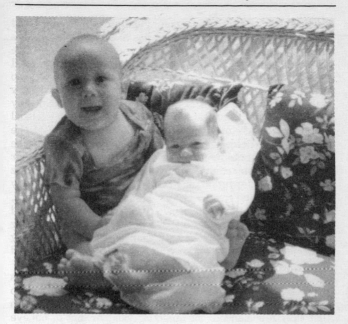

This exciting growth in eye, hand, and body control is the first major thrust of infancy. It means many things: practical concerns such as buying a bounce chair and babyproofing the house; a family "crisis" of making sure everyone gets enough sleep; and inner matters, such as the baby's mental growth and mother's occasional feelings of rejection.

Before your baby becomes really mobile and more searching, take an inventory with your husband of all the household traps the baby might fall into, and babyproof the house. Since he can already clamber out of his infant chair, a bounce chair or swing should be the next step. It should still be at a reclining angle so that even when he arches forward, the chair can support the lower half of his back. It should also be weighted at the bottom so your baby will not topple it. Because he will dream up things you might never think of, you must take precautions. Keep his chair away from heat sources such as the stove, iron, and toaster and get him a strap for his stroller.

Now that the baby can see very clearly, he can visually differentiate his parents. He may squirm, babble, and pump his arms up and down when he finds his father's or mother's face in a roomful of people. Since he can now tell which people are not his parents, his sensitivity to strangers increases. He may be particularly sensitive to strange women. When a woman "oohs" and "ahs" at him or tries to pick him up during an outing, he may voice his resentment quite clearly. Fear of strange women is often stronger than that toward strange men, probably because a woman arouses all the associations of sight, touch, smell, taste, sound, comfort, learning, and fun that the baby has had more chance to build with his mother than his father.

The baby's seeing, handling, turning, and reaching for things also help him grow aware that objects are stable and permanent, each with its own autonomy. Up to about five months of age, the baby's world is more or less a series of things that mysteriously disappear and reappear. The baby's reaching for something introduces the idea that things are beyond and apart and, therefore, separate from him. When he handles an object, he senses that its shape remains the same, even though its visual appearance changes as he turns it or as it approaches or recedes from him. He also tries to recapture objects if he loses them. For example, he leans over to look for an object he has dropped to the floor instead of simply staring at the place from which it was released. Or he will search outside his field of vision for an object he has been holding. He will play with a teddy bear, leave it for a while, and relocate it without error or hesitation. He will also anticipate a whole object by seeing only a part, and he can and does free his perception by removing minor obstacles, such as a carriage robe, from his face. But he will still give up immediately if a vanished or abandoned toy does not come readily to hand or eye. He still seems to believe that objects are alternately made and unmade. Some months later, he will realize the most amazing thing of all—things will continue to exist and happen even when they are out of hand and sight and beyond his sphere of influence. The day your baby tries to push your

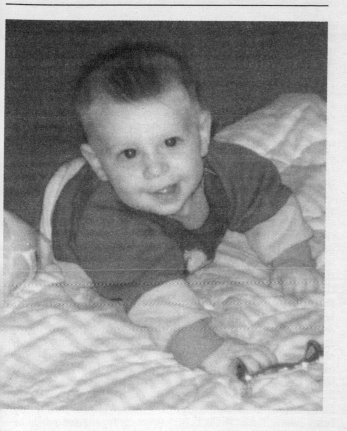

hand to make a roly-poly toy topple is the day you will know
he realizes that something or someone else besides him
makes things go.

Reaching and grabbing also help the baby grow aware
that there is a "before" and "after," a cause and effect in an
action sequence of his own making. This means he is beginning to keep track of his own actions in the immediate past.
In the next couple of months or so, your baby will know
enough about his bottle to rotate it should you hand it to him
the wrong way. He will demonstrate recognition of familiar

objects by outlining actions he habitually makes to them. The baby sees the teddy bear he likes to swing, and opens and closes his hands in an abbreviated version of the swinging movements. This body recognition is the forerunner of mature mental recognition and a first step toward baby's orienting himself to a goal.

The Family's Early Riser

All these faintly sensed but vital understandings are a lot to handle. The baby is on the brink of a great developmental surge and he actively responds to its excitements and frustrations. The average five-month-old rouses himself literally at the peep of dawn to be about this daily business of learning. The baby's four-hour sleep cycles, which crystallized at about his third month of life, make him waken about 6:00 A.M. Now, however, instead of lying quietly sucking his fist or looking at his toys, he quickly awakes to practice all his new muscular and social skills. Although he can temporarily amuse himself with rocking spread-eagled on his tummy or turning himself over, he will eventually begin to demand some attention. His crying and calling arouse the household and invite his family away from sleep to share his full day.

No parental maneuver can really impede this inner primal clock. Keeping a baby up later in the evening will not make him tired in the early morning. Feeding him at night does not help. Black shades to keep out the light that moves him are worth a try. Harnessing him to the bed may be an immediate, strong-armed answer for the desperate, but its long-range consequences are not much of a "solution" for anything. Odd as it may seem, harnessing the baby is likely to hurt his physical development less than his emotional growth. More than enough evidence from around the world suggests that physical restraint like tight swaddling only retards motor development by about a month. It is important to reinforce a baby's effort to practice and maneuver. This way you will encourage him to develop mastery over his environment.

Putting the baby farther away from the family is perhaps the kindest solution for all concerned. It not only gives you more sleep, it nudges your baby back to his own resources for a longer time.

For most babies, these antic urges spurt and ebb. But a quieter baby handles his developing awareness more subtly. Grasping and sucking on fingers, toes, and toys intensify as he lies content on his back or brings his feet to his mouth. He mouths and chews every available edge of a toy, savoring each separate fact and flavor of it. Many more active infants are happy only when they are in continuous motion— performing on their own or handled vigorously. Most free on his back, an active baby may kick against his crib mattress or the carpet and propel himself into a corner, where he wedges himself, or he may also twist his body to pull the

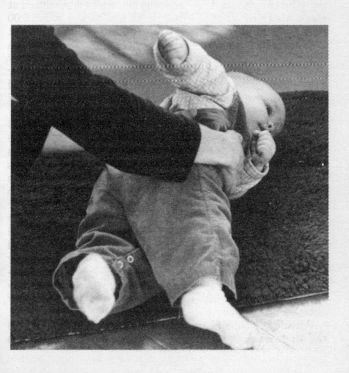

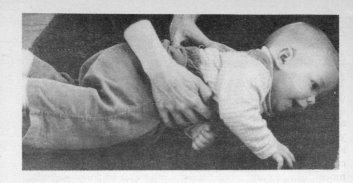

upper half over and roll onto his belly, then prop himself up on his arms, look about, and roll back again. On his tummy, desperate wriggling with his arms and legs and fierce see-sawing may also propel him. At night, a really active baby may wake several times because of the added excitement of this developmental surge. During the semi-conscious phase of his sleep cycle, he can wake up fully and try to comfort himself with activity because it is a characteristic outlet for him. Unfortunately, activity is not the solution to quieting down at nighttime.

Pinning him down with a sheet or blanket or tilting the mattress to prevent his rocking and rolling will only make him fight more furiously whenever he wakes. A late-night feeding and a short play period will release some of his energy more profitably. As little as two weeks later, you may be able to cut out your baby's nightlife.

Another way to help your baby work off some of his energy and frustration is daytime exercise sessions. You can teach your baby how to roll himself over from back to stomach. You can also show him how to calm himself as he builds to peaks of rolling. Dr. Brazelton suggests that you "flatten the baby on his tummy and bring his thumb to his mouth. Then hold him." The baby may be outraged at first with your intrusion, but eventually he should begin to quiet during the practice sessions and later during the night if he has learned what you mean. This kind of assertive yet loving intervention contrasts sharply with more forceful restraint. Insistent or tactless teaching efforts can assault an infant's sensitivity and cut his desire to learn for himself.

Serious Language Study

You would think that with all this energy devoted to physical development, your baby would have no time for anything else. Not at all. This is the month your baby obviously starts serious "language study." As you may have guessed from your own experience with your baby, expressive language starts not with the first word, but with his first use of cries to attract attention. Scientists agree that at about one month of age, and even earlier according to some parents, infant cries of discomfort, pain and hunger can be discriminated by the listener. In the next few months, cooing, squeals of delight, scolding, and grunts of disgust clearly show his reactions to situations. The gesture language of looking and reaching is yet another pipeline of communication between parent and baby. As usual, a baby will approach these efforts in characteristic style. Keep in mind that not all infants are equally interested in speech. The earlier babblers may be the talkers, the ones disposed toward language and that kind of interaction. Some of the "talkers" will screech for the sheer pleasure of experimenting with their sound equipment, while others display a subtle and varied register of tone, quiet trilling, and volume control. Silent babies may be too busy sizing up their world to spend much time "talking" about it. Quiet ones may digest and explore speech and other sounds more privately. An

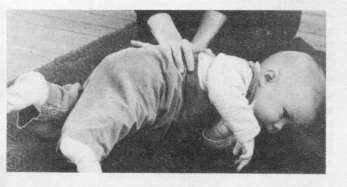

acoustically sensitive baby may, for example, combine listening adventure with producing sounds—his own or mechanical ones. The tinkle of a bell-toy can hold him spellbound. He may even learn to turn it so that it makes different tones. If he prefers to control and produce slight changes in sound himself, the drawn-out variations of a music box may be less absorbing. This combination of extrasensitive hearing and tone production are basics of good musicianship, so keep an ear out if your baby shows these attributes.

Most babies will communicate with anyone who is available. Your baby will probably watch mouths, jaws, and faces as people make sounds to him, then experiment with his own vocal and facial movements. The consonants *p*, *b*, and *m*, made with the lips, are the first sounds a baby makes. The next consonants that an infant learns, *t*, *d*, and *n*, are formed with the gums and teeth. Hence, it is hardly surprising that the earliest words babies speak include *papa*, *dada*, *baba*, *mama*, *nana*, and *tata*. When a five-month-old produces a chain of rhythmic, syllable-like sounds; "da-da-da," "ma-ma-ma," "ba-ba-ba," many parents and grandparents think that the baby is tagging them. It is more likely that he is merely playing with his vocal organs. Vowels, such as "ah-ah-ah" and "ee-ee-oo," are the primary sounds babbled during the fifth month. As his babbling increases, the baby's sounds become more and more controlled. You can encourage his babbling by reacting to it quickly with your verbal response and smiles.

Since feedback may be one of the most important elements in early speech learning, a baby's family should always respond to him. *Dada* repeatedly brings father, and *bye-bye* prompts delighted squeals from his sister. Even though he cannot associate sequences of sounds with their word meanings yet, he learns to imitate himself and to repeat what were originally trial-and-error combinations to get the expected response. A pattern of joyful exchange set, the baby will also try to imitate the inflections in your voice and move on to more and more complex language successes.

Besides encouraging this important practice and its companion, a feeling of mastery, this reinforcement has even

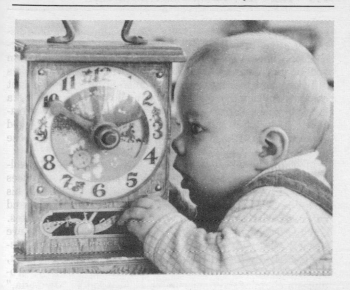

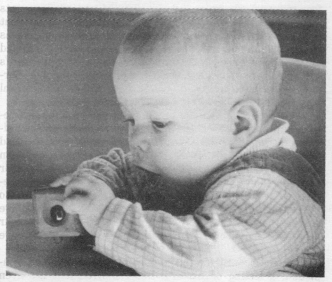

more specific teaching functions. The identification of people and objects is based on the general principle of naming. Once acquired, it lays the entire foundation of a human being's ability to symbolize. If you have listened carefully to your baby, you will quickly realize that at first most of his sounds are not those of any language, let alone English. Sometimes the baby will also use sounds like a guttural *r* or nasalized "vowels" that are really more appropriate to German and French. As English-speakers, mother and father generally respond to the sounds that seem most like those of English and, of course, their sounds, which are English, are models for their baby. In response to this selective reinforcement, the baby's non-English sounds very gradually, almost imperceptibly drop out. Many months later, your toddler will have a system of real English sounds. Do not expect perfect English. More than three-quarters of your tot's speech sounds will be clear by the time he is two, but there is an important difference between understandable English *sounds* and understandable English. The distribution of vowels to consonants is also very important. Only by about two and a half will this distribution approximate that of an adult. What is more, the sound system of English is only one of three major aspects of language your youngster is going to learn. The other two are its vocabulary and grammar.

Social Uses of Early Language

A baby will deliberately use his newly found vocal skills to intrude upon your attentions to other things so you will focus them where he thinks they should be—on him. He may start to smile and vocalize to a visiting friend. When this does not stop her chattering, he may twist around and try to divert. If this fails, you may be stunned and amused to find your baby babbling more and more loudly. To continue your conversation, you may have to remove him from your lap or to another room. Do not be intimidated if the baby suddenly disintegrates into frantic activity or crying. These conversational exchanges are still a great effort for him. Your interaction is as important as your fear of "teaching" him beyond his endurance. Human stimulation of infant sounds is vital. Research with infants born to deaf parents indicates that before six months of age, parental inability to hear and imitate an infant's sounds hardly influences their quality. Their cooing and babbling are very much like those of babies with parents who can hear. But later the lack of response and the differences in his parents' sounds start to influence those of the baby. They lose intonation and grow nasal in quality. Conversely, a hearing loss handicaps a child so much that he can behave autistically— out of touch with his environment. He may have a faraway look in his eyes and withdraw into repetitive, self-stimulating habits to fill the deficit of stimulation from the outside world.

One of the major handicaps of institutionalized toddlers and educationally deprived youngsters is their inability to communicate. Dr. Bettye Caldwell ascribes this to lack of language stimulation. The infant's caretakers have neither the time nor often the interest to talk to him. During the first year of life, there *is* a natural unfolding of language and physical events that the environment can speed or delay, but never reorder. We cannot, for example, teach a baby to utter prepositional phrases before he babbles. The important thing is to talk to your baby.

The fostering of speech begins with the parents' encouraging, affectionate sounds and gestures as she or he feeds, bathes, and makes the baby comfortable. Even at two months, it is more important for a baby to direct his smiling and vocalizing to a responsive face. Speech thus becomes associated in the baby's mind with identification, comfort, and communication. Later, accompanying words with actions, like *all gone* and *up-and-off;* inventing naming games involving baby's nose, toes, feet, hands, and mouth; and singing to him and repeating nursery rhymes can all help to make speech interesting and pleasant. A home that provides a palate of occasional sounds—a chiming grandfather clock, a music box, bell-toys, or chirping birds, without a confusing blare of background noise—helps to make an infant aware of different sound qualities.

More on Baby Talk

Language specialists are not in agreement as to whether or not parents should speak baby talk to their infants and very young children. Some think it impedes the development of normal language; others believe that baby talk provides practice in producing sounds. Although speaking in baby talk may not be harmful early on, its use after the earliest years of life may keep a child's speech locked in at an infantile level. At this stage, don't worry about baby talk. Use it if you wish. Every known language community in the world, admittedly or not, provides this special form of its language to its infant members precisely to teach them to communicate. Your baby's word approximations, a normal and necessary aspect of vocabulary development, need not be paragons of precision. Only the number of words attempted should increase. The baby just needs to hear sounds and human speech.

Unneeded, Unwanted, and Unloved

About the fifth or sixth month, many mothers say they feel left out. As their babies become more competent physically, they see the end of their child's need for mother despite the reality that his need will continue for many years. Overreacting to the baby's relative independence is easy. Two kinds of separations by which mothers express these inner feelings are weaning, if they are breast-feeding, and returning to work.

Weaning

If you are breast-feeding your baby, you may rationalize weaning in many ways—all justifiable. He is eating enough solids so that he needs only three feedings anyway. With a bottle, other family members can feed him if you are particularly busy. You will not be as tired when you relinquish this extra physical drain. (Unfortunately, nursing can add to a mother's fatigue.) The baby calls you all day and holds out his arms to be picked up when he sees you. His unanswered appeals make you feel guilty, although you "know"

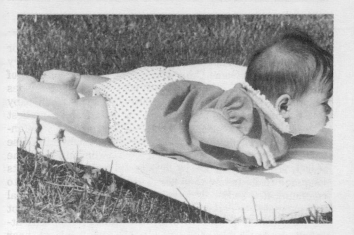

that his frustration when you do not always respond can push him positively toward self-sufficiency. Or the baby himself seems disinterested in nursing.

Do not get so wrapped up in your feelings toward your baby that you forget that other mothers and babies are caught up in the same things you are; that they also are experiencing this vast sequence of events and growth. Actually your baby may be showing the first of three major lags in an infant's interest in breast-feeding. According to Dr. Brazelton: "This one is generally associated with the sudden widening, visual interest in his surroundings. The second accompanies the tremendous motor spurt of seven months. The third occurs between nine and twelve months." A few babies never lose interest and probably have to be pushed away. When a baby begins to lose interest after nine months, taking him up on it seems appropriate in our culture. He has had enough nutritional sucking and probably does not really need more.

Many mothers around the world nurse children for several years to give them antibodies against disease, as well as the protein, calcium, and vitamins they would not get otherwise, to protect them as best they can from the incredibly high rates of infant deaths in many developing nations. The natural cycle of conception, pregnancy, birth, and lactation is virtually unbroken until menopause. In our culture, the merits of breast-feeding for the baby's health decrease as he matures. As long as the mother nurses, her baby accrues the benefits of immunity to some diseases and allergies. But after the initial start, they are not necessary to his survival. The benefit of nursing for the mother's health may be a different matter.

There are studies currently going on to assess the incidence of breast cancer amongst mothers who have nursed their babies versus those who have not. There is presently nothing conclusive about the data being collected.

If you really want to, you can wean your baby in a week, because your milk will decrease as stimulation drops. However, weaning is more traumatic for mothers than many think. Besides the emotional jolt, a shorter, less intense version of postpartum depression may set in due to hormonal changes.

A slow, gradual weaning gives you and your infant an opportunity to adjust. If you choose this alternative, pediatricians recommend dropping the noon feeding first, the evening feeding next, and the early-morning feeding last. Late night and early morning are peaceful times free of the noises of daytime or the distractions of other children. Whether you wean now or later, the early-morning feeding is usually the hardest one to relinquish, especially if you are used to nursing and cuddling your baby in bed and then putting him back in his crib so you can grab a precious extra hour of sleep.

Some babies, perhaps yours included, appear to suck their fingers more after they are weaned. At this stage, the extra sucking probably reflects tension before a burst of physical growth rather than upset from the weaning.

Having seen their babies through their difficult first months, many mothers consider returning to work. They have to weigh the balance between their needs and their infants' need for a dependable nurturing figure.

A baby learns so many fundamentals between three and twelve months of life that he is especially vulnerable to intellectual deprivation if his environment lacks sufficient stimulation and encouragement. A consistent substitute caregiver needs to be involved in the baby's mental, physical, and social progress, even to the point of getting down on his hands and knees, if necessary, and showing the baby how to back down the stairs when he is learning to get around instead of parking him in a playpen or stuffing him with food.

A baby may react to his mother's absence, whether parceled out in nine-to-five packets or prolonged indefinitely, by crying a lot, reaching out to people, refusing food, forgetting his latest physical accomplishments, clinging when you come home, and fearing strangers even more than usual.

At the same time, the baby whose mother returns to him every day will be able to carry an image of her in his mind, and even anticipate her return, thanks to his improving memory. When you do find a competent substitute caregiver for your baby, let him (and your older children, if you have them) get to know the person in advance.

If a young mother needs help in identifying and moderating her complex feelings at this juncture, her baby's pediatrician can be a great resource. If you do not have a pediatrician who can offer guidance and understanding, you might try to find one who can.

Weaning is the transition from sucking to get food from the breast or a bottle to feeding from a cup or a spoon. Psychoanalyst Hiag Akmakjian says, "It is a mistake to think of weaning as 'taking away' the breast or bottle. Much more positively, weaning means introducing a baby to new foods and a new method of eating. It is a step forward, not a deprivation."

There is no definite time when the physical and emotional benefits of breast-feeding or the sucking and nutritional satisfaction of bottle-feeding suddenly cease for all babies. Many authorities suggest that a sensible time to wean to the bottle is at about three months. Others maintain that the sucking needs of babies normally diminish somewhere between six and ten months. Of course, weaning may need to be done earlier in the case of working mothers. In any event, it is difficult for a baby for whom this is all-important to be weaned overnight. It also is advisable not to start weaning during any time of special physical or emotional stress; for example, teething, extremely hot weather, when parents go away on a vacation, or for other reasons.

WHEN TO WEAN FROM THE BREAST

The ideal time to wean a baby is when he is ready for it; that is, when he begins decidedly to lose interest in breast-feeding. In general, that can be anytime after his sixth month. If your baby consistently turns away, cries, or pushes away bottle or cup, he probably is not ready for weaning from your breast. However, just as a baby should not be taken out of the sucking phase too soon, it is not advisable to let him stay in it too long, because that would work against his developing independence. When some emergency makes sudden weaning from the breast necessary, it is important to consult your pediatrician about the proper formula to substitute.

WEANING TO A BOTTLE

If the mother has been breast-feeding and no longer wants to do so, it would do no harm to switch to a bottle for one of the baby's meals each day, increasing that later to two or three bottles a day. However, the change must be made gradually. Your baby will probably object to the bottle the first few times.

Usually it is easier to get breast-fed babies to accept a bottle if they have already grown used to an occasional or a daily relief bottle. They will then take more readily to full-time bottle-feeding. The following are some helpful hints about bottle weaning: (1) Start by offering your baby part of a single feeding from a bottle, giving him time to get used to the feel and taste of a rubber nipple and the different taste of the milk; (2) Gradually increase the amount of formula until he has taken one entire feeding by bottle for several days; (3) When your baby is adjusted to one complete bottle feeding per day, apply the same gradual process to another feeding, and so on, until the weaning has been accomplished.

Your baby should get lots of cuddling, stroking, and encouragement to make up for the lost skin-to-skin contact.

WEANING TO A CUP

Theoretically, if you wean from breast to cup, you can save an extra step (the bottle), but in practice this sometimes proves more difficult. Most mothers introduce a bottle occasionally to get the baby used to something other than the breast, just in case they cannot be present for a particular feeding. The occasional bottle can contain water.

Some babies begin voluntarily to drink from a cup because they see their parents (or older siblings) doing so and are ready for it. In general, breast-fed babies appear to accept a cup before they are a year old, while some bottle-fed babies are ready only as late as in their second year. You may find the suggestions below helpful:

1. Experiment once in a while, starting when your baby is four or five months old, to see whether he will willingly take a few sips from a cup.

2. A nonbreakable baby cup with two handles and fitted with a spout is recommended. Give your baby a small, nonbreakable, brightly colored cup of his own to play with.

3. When you give your baby a cup to drink from, drink from a cup yourself. Imitation is the most natural way for babies to learn.

4. Expect spilling when your baby tries to lift the cup himself (most babies cannot completely manipulate a cup until they are about one and a half years old).

5. Your baby will probably object less to the introductory sips coming from a strange new object if it contains water rather than milk.

6. At first, offer only small sips of milk, gradually working up to the usual amount for one feeding.

7. When a complete feeding is being taken happily from the cup, gradually replace any breast or bottle feedings in the same manner, one by one. The weaning process may take weeks or a few months.

8. Force of any kind prolongs weaning (whether it is deliberate withholding of breast or bottle or subtle coaxing).

After you completely stop breast-feeding, your production of breast milk will cease quickly. If your breasts should become engorged, you may relieve your discomfort by expressing milk for the first two or three days. Your doctor can show you how to empty your breasts by hand. One way is to place the pads of your thumb and forefinger on opposite sides of your breast, about one and a half inches from your nipple. Remember not to touch your nipple. Then press deeply into your breast and establish a steady rhythm of pressing and releasing your grip. You will attain skill after some practice. You may wish instead to use a breast pump, which is available in most drugstores. Limiting your fluid intake or wearing a breast binder may also be helpful. Your discomfort should end within a week.

Working Mothers

To work or not to work outside the home while children are very young is the difficult question that faces many mothers, and increasing numbers of mothers are choosing employment. Statistics show that more than 50 percent of children in the United States have working mothers at this point in time. For many, there is no choice; their income must supplement or completely support the family; for others, it is a question of personal preference. A major consideration is whether the mother's salary will cover the costs she incurs. First, there is the expense of child care and help with the housework. Skilled day-care workers cannot be had for a song. If you are counting on a day-care center to play substitute mother while you work, keep in mind that good day care is costly.

After careful consideration of the financial aspects, a mother needs to review her reasons for wanting to go to work. Would she be happier working outside her home? Does she wish to return to a professional field in which she felt competent and satisfied? Or does she desire to escape the seemingly endless chores at home that she finds repetitive, uncreative, and boring?

In *Three Years to Grow*, Sara D. Gilbert says: "If a mother must or strongly wants to work outside the home, there is no reason why, for the baby's sake, she shouldn't, as long as she plans for his needs with the same loving, intelligent interest she would give those needs if she were at home."

Of course, the foremost consideration should be the baby's requirement for a suitable caregiver. An appropriate, consistent substitute should fill in the hours not covered by the parents. Pediatricians and child psychologists agree that there must be one dependable person for the baby to rely on for the attachment, affection, comfort, and learning that are his due. The substitute caregiver should be concerned not only with the baby's physical well-being, but also with his mental, psychological, and social progress. A baby learns so many fundamentals during the first twelve months of his life that it is essential for the parent-substitute to be warm and loving and have sufficient training and ability to further the baby's language acquisition, general learning, and his building of a positive self-image.

There are various possibilities for good child care. One obvious choice is the father. A nurturing father's feelings of self-esteem are as invested in his children and his ability to be a loving parent as in his work and career. If he is self-

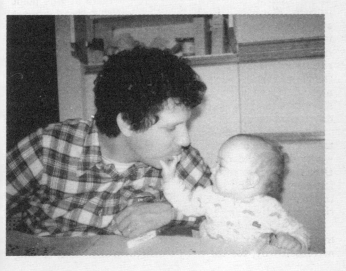

employed or has a flexible work schedule or would prefer taking care of his children, the child-care problem may be solved.

Present-day participation of fathers in childbirth classes and at the delivery appears to be creating closer involvement with their wives and their babies. Fathers who are caring husbands and are on hand for their children truly enrich and bless the lives of their families. Besides supporting their families financially, they spend considerable time and energy on some part of the day-to-day chores child care and running a household entail. Such fathers let their wives know that they value everything their wives do for them and their children. Nonetheless, in all but a small number of families, today's working mothers still assume major responsibility in the home.

Grandparents can sometimes be counted on to provide loving child care. However, they might not be a good choice if they strongly disapprove of the mother's working or they criticize the parents' methods of child-rearing.

There are several kinds of child-care possibilities in addition to mother or father at home; for example, a nanny; an au pair girl or a baby-sitter in the home; a family day-care home; or a day-care center where the ratio of babies to staff is no more than four to one. Choosing the best substitute care requires your getting informed about child development, appreciating the characteristics of your baby, and knowing exactly what each setting offers. There are particular advantages and disadvantages in each setup for different children at different ages.

Day care for infants is available in some communities, but there can be long waiting lists. Sometimes the working mother can find a woman who enjoys child care and homemaking and is willing to care for another baby in addition to her own.

Children appear to be better off with satisfied, relaxed substitute caregivers and happy, part-time mothers than full-time, frustrated ones. The most discontented women are mothers who feel trapped and lonely at home, and wish they could be employed.

The Working Mother and Breast-Feeding

In early infancy, from birth to seven months of age, infants thrive on love, comforting, and good basic care that satisfy their physical and emotional needs. Working mothers should not feel guilty about leaving their three-month-olds who are easily comforted and have settled into a predictable daily routine of feeding, eliminating, and nap times.

From seven to twelve months, when stranger anxiety normally occurs, your baby may suddenly be reluctant to stay with anyone outside his family. If possible, parents should not start substitute child care during this period.

If they so desire, women can continue to breast-feed their babies after returning to work. They can breast-feed before leaving in the morning and at the day's end, and use prepared infant formula for the other feedings.

For working mothers who choose not to continue breast-feeding their babies, infant formula manufacturers are constantly improving their products in an effort to approximate the composition of human milk. Commercial formulas are available in powders and concentrates that need to be mixed with water, and prepared formulas that do not require dilution. Of course, the latter are more costly.

Parents need to read all formula labels with care. Soy-based or other specialized formulas are available for babies with lactose intolerance or an allergy to cow's milk. Your doctor can help you select the formula that will be best for your baby. Parents often assume that their infants prefer warm liquids. Actually, infants like formula or expressed breast milk at body or room temperature. All liquids and other foods need to be temperature-tested before they are fed to infants.

All mothers, fathers, and other caregivers who bottle-feed need to spend time holding and cuddling the baby during feedings. The positive bonding and sense of security that result from this interchange are essential to every baby's well-being.

Progress Report

FEEDING

Feeding periods are more enjoyable now, although messy. Your baby is becoming more interested and cooperative. He has established a definite interval between feeding and elimination. Even less adaptable babies have stopped the late-night feedings by themselves. Most can probably give up the 10 P.M. feeding as well. Of course, you may still want that chance for special closeness with your baby, particularly if other children prevent peaceful daytime feedings.

EATING IS PLAY

Feeding sessions are opportunities for socializing. If you talk to your baby during feedings, his cooing, gurgling, and vocalizing will last for as long as thirty minutes before he returns to breast or bottle to finish. A social animal with none of our social conventions, your baby relishes his role as the sloppy prince. He always has sucked his fingers after a bite, but now he may try his entire fist, or prefer to play with his father's hands while he is feeding him. His delicate licking of lips and fingers does not quite clean his hand to prevent smearing his face. He is so anxious to "talk," to look at his family in action, or to play with your hair, face, or clothes that he sucks in short bursts or stops entirely, drooling milk down his cheeks and chin. Although drooling, finger-sucking, exploration of his mouth with his hand, and shortened interest in the breast or bottle may indicate teething, all signal your baby's broadening interest in his world.

The baby's reduction of nursing time in favor of people-watching is no problem for him. If he is breast-feeding, he may be able to take what he needs from your breasts in the first five minutes. However, you may have a problem. Stimulation to the breasts, cut abruptly, can decrease your milk supply. If this happens, more frequent nursing will bring it back. Another help might be morning and evening feedings in a dark, quiet room with no distractions. Your baby should suck for the usual period and then your milk will return. You might also try this if shortening a feeding is necessary or if your baby is not eating enough.

Despite the baby's distractibility and the inconveniences, feeding times with the family should be retained whenever possible, because they are among your baby's most valuable socializing periods. After all, your delightful dynamo is well worth the effort. Dr. Leon Yarrow, of the National Institutes of Health, says that a baby who lives during his first six months in an environment charged with frequent, exuberant expressions of good feelings and lots of face-to-face socializing with loved ones will have far more than the usual share of social initiative and get-up-and-go.

SLEEPING

After your baby is a couple of months old, you may begin to see his preference for a certain sleeping position, either on his tummy or his back. Some parents try to change this urge in their babies because they may have read that one position may tend to flatten the head or another may not be good for the legs or feet. Most pediatricians believe that it is much more important for parents to satisfy their infant's natural inclination to repeat a comfortable pattern in sleep than to worry about some of the pros and cons that are presented for each sleep position.

If your baby's head starts to flatten from his keeping it to one side, there are some things you can do to get him to turn his head to both sides. If you alternate putting him to bed with his head at the foot and the head of the crib and there is a particular thing he likes to look at, he will turn his head in that direction part of the time. You can attach some toys or bright things to the crib in such a way that your baby has to turn his head to look at them. Incidentally, head flattening corrects itself in due course. You will also find that after your baby learns to roll over, his sleeping position will tend to change.

During the night, infants enter a semi-conscious, semialert state during which they talk, cry out, or move around, and after which they have to get themselves back to sleep. It is a good idea for you to let your baby do this by himself lest your presence become a routine part of his pattern of resuming sleep.

NAPS

At about the fifth month, babies are generally taking two or three naps a day. This usually depends upon whether or not the baby is getting a 10 P.M. bottle. Some babies have a short morning nap and a long afternoon nap, or vice versa, or a morning and an afternoon nap of about the same length of time. Sleep is very individual and, of course, varies from time to time. For example, a new tooth coming in may make a baby fretful or wake him up from a nap.

By the time a baby approaches his first birthday, he is going through the transitional period of giving up one of his two daytime naps. You may have to delay the morning naptime by giving your baby an early lunch, then putting him down, and upon his waking, giving him some more

---

Helpful Pointers on Sleeping

1. Do not pick your baby up after he has been tucked in for the night to exhibit him to company.

2. It is not a good idea to take your infant out in the evening. Good sleeping patterns cannot be established unless a baby is put to bed every night at about the same time. Try to find a reliable baby-sitter or a cooperative baby-sitting pool in your neighborhood.

3. Never leave your baby alone in the house whether he is asleep or awake.

4. Do not let your baby go to sleep with a bottle, because the nipple left in a baby's mouth while sleeping may cause malformed jaws and poor dental development.

5. Another good reason for a regular bedtime is that when babies go to bed later than usual, they generally do not make up their missed sleep by awaking later in the morning.

If you have any questions about your baby's sleep positions or behavior, talk to your pediatrician.

lunch. That way he may be able to last until suppertime. (Just having a morning nap tends to make a baby fussy by midafternoon and too tired to eat supper.)

There is a time in a baby's life when one nap is too little and two naps are too much. This can be a trying period for your baby and you. However, with gentle prodding you can steer him toward the afternoon nap by being patient, giving him the earlier lunch, and putting him to bed at night just a bit earlier than usual.

Some babies go to sleep almost immediately after being placed in their cribs. However, there are others who seem to need to cry or fret before they can release themselves to sleep. A few others may talk to themselves or bang around in their cribs before they drop off. When you put your baby down for a nap, see that he is comfortable and leave him. He has to learn to get himself to sleep.

Of course, if your baby cries for any length of time, you will want to check him. Perhaps you need to help him burp up a bubble, or another diaper change may be in order. The baby who knows you mean it when you say good night is really more comfortable about bed than the one who feels he ought to put up a fuss just to see what you will do next.

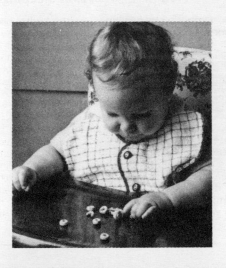

THE FIFTH MONTH

Motor Development	Language
### Gross Motor	### Vocalizing

Gross Motor

On tummy, lifts head and chest high off mattress. On back, lifts head and shoulders. Brings feet to mouth and sucks on toes.

Vigorous activity of all limbs.

Lies on tummy, arms and legs extended. On tummy, rocks like an airplane, limbs extended and back arched. Rolls from back to side. Rolls from stomach to back. On tummy, pushes on hands and draws up knees. May locomote by rocking, rolling, and twisting; or on back, by kicking against flat surface.

Easily pulled to stand. When supported under arms, stands and moves body up and down; stamps one foot then the other.

Sitting

Sits supported for long periods (thirty minutes); back firm.

Seated or pulled to sit, holds and balances head steady and erect continuously. Helps in pulling up body, flexes head forward, flexes trunk, draws legs toward tummy. Seated, can grasp object.

Sits alone momentarily.

Fine Motor

Plays with rattle placed in hands. May hold bottle, one or two hands.

Reaches for ring and grasps; aim good.

Vocalizing

Utters vowel sounds—"ee," "ay," "ey," "ah," "ooh"—and a few consonantlike sounds, *d, b, l, m.* Vocalizes spontaneously to himself; to toys.

May babble to gain attention.

Watches mouths closely; experiments with own sounds after hearing others. Tries to imitate inflections.

Strong drive to experiment with own sounds, especially when there is saliva in mouth. Listens intently to sounds.

Responding

Responds to human sounds more definitively; turns head, seems to look for speaker. Understands name.

Mental	Social

Mental

Sensory Response

Learning to identify mother's voice through its sound qualities.

Attention Span

Alert up to an hour and a half to two hours. Looks about in new situations. Turns head deliberately to sound or to follow vanishing object.

Eye-Hand Coordination

Eyes cooperate in grasping and manipulation. Raises hand in vicinity of an object; alternately glances between hand and object; gradually closes gap and grasps. Picks up block on contact. Reaches for object with two hands from sides to middle of his body, sometimes with closed fists. Hands may meet below, beyond, or in front of object.

Wants to touch, hold, turn, shake, mouth, taste objects.

Visually searches for fast-moving objects and for objects he has looked away from. Leans over to look for fallen object. Removes from face minor obstacles to vision.

Memory

Anticipates a whole object by seeing only a part.

Recognizes familiar objects. Remembers his own actions in the immediate past.

Has mental model for human face. Discriminates parents and sibs from others. May resent strangers, particularly women.

Social

Personal

Shows fear, disgust, anger.

Discriminates self and parent in mirror. Smiles and vocalizes to mirror image. May bang playfully.

Makes faces in imitation.

Interaction

Smiles to human faces and voices. May distinguish familiar and unfamiliar adults. Smiles or vocalizes to make social contact.

Shows happiness in presence of other people, especially parents. Enjoys prolonged interaction with adults—game play, singing, giggling, tickling, exchanging smiles and sounds with parents.

Shows anticipation, waves and raises arms to be picked up. Tries to get close to person near crib. Clings when held.

May learn to tease. Vocalizes to interrupt others' conversation. Stops crying when talked to.

Expresses protest—resists adult who tries to take toy.

Cries when someone leaves him.

Cultural Self-Help/Routines

Interest in breast-feeding lags. Takes solids well. May start on cup.

Alert at least half of waking hours.

Wakes promptly at dawn.

(continued)

THE FIFTH MONTH *(cont.)*

Motor Development	Language
Swaps objects from hand to hand. Grabs or waves object with either hand.	
Skills of handling, reaching, fisting, etc., now tried out on objects.	

Please do not regard this chart as a rigid timetable. Babies are unpredictable. Some perform an activity earlier or later than the chart indicates.

Mental	Social
Deliberately and systematically imitates sounds and movements.	**Play and Playthings**

Mental

Deliberately and systematically imitates sounds and movements.

Body and Object Awareness

Interacts with mirrors and well-designed crib objects. Gradual emergence of capacity to use hands as reaching tools under guidance of vision; brings hands together at mid-stomach; explores clothing, etc. Explores visually. Rears head to peer about.

Tries to maintain through repetition an interesting change in his environment.

Discriminating and Associating

Holds one block, regards second. Drops first to take second.

Social

Play and Playthings

Frolics when played with. Plays with rattle; pats bottle or breast.

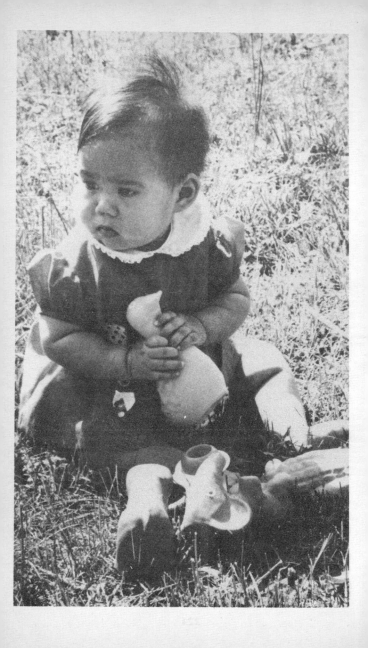

The Sixth Month

SITTING PRETTY

The world of the six-month-old has truly become a sitting-up world that he can handle, "talk" with, and play in. Visually alert almost half his waking hours, he can sit for long stretches in a bounce chair and play with toys for at least two hours. In his chair, he can visually follow objects at many different distances and speeds. He can crane over to reach and look at his feet or reconnoiter the surrounding territory. He can bounce over to intriguing objects, reach for anything he sees, and look at anything he manages to grab. This apparent mania to look and grab accurately is critical to your baby's awareness of things in his environment, even though it may seem that all your good decorative art will be demolished.

Your baby can probably sit and balance well by himself for approximately half an hour. He can even balance on an adult's shoulders, holding onto his friend's head for support. The gradual appearance of a straight back as he sits and as you gently pull him up to sit reflects a slow downward extension of muscular control. His hands will also tell you how new his sitting skill is. Even after he can sit alone, a baby will use his hands and arms for balance. When your baby manipulates a toy as he sits unsupported, you will know he has become secure in his prowess.

Although he still has to be helped to sit, he can occasionally roll into a near-sitting posture by bending himself in the middle as he rolls. Some very active infants can already get themselves to sit if they get into a crawl position, sit back on their legs, and stick them out in front.

A six-month-old can also arch his back and look upside down at things, twist in all directions, roll, flop, and creep. Dressing him may become a judo contest in which you ply him with a series of toys, each of which works for only a short time. In preparation for crawling, the first effective way to get around, a baby will inefficiently worm his way across a room by twisting and rolling. You may have to constantly extract him from under furniture.

A baby this age may also crouch on his hands and knees and hurtle himself forward, only to splatter as he flops with outspread limbs. He may aim a series of flops at a desirable object, which can mysteriously disappear under his body if he overshoots his target. Some babies can even creep with their tummies pressed to the ground, pushing with their feet and steering with outstretched arms. It is unlike crawling, which features bent knees and elbows.

In both flopping and creeping, a baby often goes backward first. Although he may try to move forward, he cannot count on his sense of direction yet. He will go backward more often than forward. Only after quite some time will this reverse.

The early decision in favor of forward instead of backward propulsion must partly depend on a developing awareness that forward is faster. Nature is no help at this point either, because the muscles that enable forward direction are still not as strong as those that push him backward.

Many babies love to stand or be stood up at this age, supported by their parents or holding onto objects. In their infant chairs, they can stand with substantial support. At first, your baby may practice holding on. As he grows competent, he may support himself with only one hand and hold up the other.

A very few six-month-olds will insist on moving from one spot holding onto your hands. Although this generally doesn't happen until about the ninth month, your baby may grunt or fuss at you until you let him go somewhere. With one, then the other stiffened leg, he will swing out like a tiny robot, body rigid and face puckered as he concentrates all energy on his new task. Of course, he's on his way toward real walking.

Dr. Brazelton notes that the remarkable energy flow in an infant's long practice hours "can hardly be reproduced by an adult. Jim Thorpe, the famous four-star athlete, is said to have imitated each move in a baby's active day. He gave out, exhausted, after four hours. The infant continued for eight or more." The infant's relentless practice of his sensory, physical, and mental abilities, in fact, testifies that the need to learn is at least as important as pleasure-seeking in determining behavior during the first two years of life.

Speaking Out

Just as locomotion is a way to get about in physical space, language is a way to get about in the social world. It allows a person to express his wants and influence the people around him. The sequence of motor and language events in your baby's life are so universal that you can pretty much predict where the baby is at in his language learning from what he's practicing physically. Although a six-month-old's vocal efforts may dwindle while he practices physical tasks, verbal expressiveness and continuous babbling are the order of the day. He can grunt or complain when he gets into difficulty, coo or gurgle with quiet pleasure, squeal with excitement, giggle in play, chortle with self-satisfaction, belly-laugh with power, growl or fuss with frustration. He can vary the volume, pitch, and rate of his babbling.

Babbling—long strings of vowels loosely connected with consonants—is among the first real signs of language growth. It is so gratifying to a baby that he'll practice his interminable strings with or without benefit of an approving audience. He loves to hear his own voice.

For girls, babbling seems a sign of mental competence. Baby girls who babble to faces and vocalize often in testing situations tend to be more attentive and obtain higher intelligence scores as toddlers and as adults than those who vocalize less. Possibly, scientists speculate, girls are "wired" to verbalize more when an interesting event captures their attention. Perhaps infant vocalization scores better predict future I.Q. for girls because their overall rate of mental development is more stable. No one really knows yet.

Your baby's babbling repertoire may include "ga-ga-ga" or "ba-ba-ba." When his brother ignores him, he may call something close to his brother's name. Of course, since his parents are the most important people in his world, he is very likely to say *Dada* and call *Mama*. *Dada*, one of the first infant vocalizations, is linked quickly to diversion and fun. Since mother means business, feeding, and relief of difficulty, *Mama* may be voiced at first with overtones of complaint. Even when he's not in trouble, he may call you "for the hell of it." As you rush to avert disaster, you may find him safely on his back, pleased at your appearance. Don't be angry. He is just practicing his skill in naming and calling loved ones. It is important that he try out his power over the world.

Babies who have learned to expect a response from their environment trust it and are more flexible than those who have called and cried in vain too often. Babies in a nursery with few adults adapt much more slowly to a regular daily feeding schedule and night sleep when they are shifted to one caretaker than babies who have had one-to-one care all along. These babies have learned that they can expect regularity in response to their initiative. By calling you, the baby has learned to strip down to a very neat signal the behavior that brings your rewarding appearance.

As your baby learns to make sounds, still mostly vowel-like, his appreciation of other sounds will increase. Music may excite him so much that he will babble more, hum, sway, or bounce rhythmically in his chair.

Human speech, especially mother's voice, is a very important part of a baby's sound environment. By this time, it has already acquired significance. Any sound will temporarily stop a baby's babbling as he listens to it. Music stops the baby's vocalizing longest. But voices make the baby pay attention hardest, and only voices make the baby babble more after his initial pause. Babies also babble back most to female voices. The baby is not only differentiating male from female, he is also responding appropriately to his experience. Who, after all, has been his constant language teacher, other than mother?

Recent research at Harvard's Center for Cognitive Studies indicates that talking to a baby is crucial to mental growth. In a study using the familiar peekaboo game, a four-month-old baby watched a rubber toy appear and disappear. Its reappearance was sometimes silent, sometimes marked by its own squeak, sometimes by mother's speech. Her voice was the only condition that reliably produced the baby's smile of recognition. Silent reappearance of the object never did. Research also indicates that even a two-month-old is quite able to associate sound with its source, and he can grow very disturbed at any change in production, location, or volume. The localization in space of a sound guides the infant's *visual* attention to the information source. Sound stops and highlights the relatively continuous flow of the visual world. Language plays an important role in skillful development of attention, perhaps *the* critical mental accomplishment of the first year of life.

Formation of Teeth

Tooth formation begins in the fetus in the early months of pregnancy. A balanced, nutritious diet is a prerequisite for strong, healthy teeth. The first two baby teeth to erupt are usually the lower central incisors. The average baby is six months old when he gets his first tooth; seven months old when his second lower incisor erupts, but he has been drooling, biting, and having periods of fretfulness from the age of three or four months.

Teething can cause crankiness and irritability. The baby wants to bite on any and all objects he can find. The gums may be sore. An ice cube wrapped in a damp cloth may help to ease the pain. Babies also like to chew on slices of raw apple, carrot and celery sticks, and dry toast, as well as chilled, hard rubber teething rings. Pediatricians do not recommend paregoric today, the traditional remedy, because it contains a narcotic.

Many teething babies have diarrhea, which is caused by the extra production of saliva that overdigests the baby's food. Give your baby plenty of fluids to counteract any loss from dehydration that diarrhea can cause.

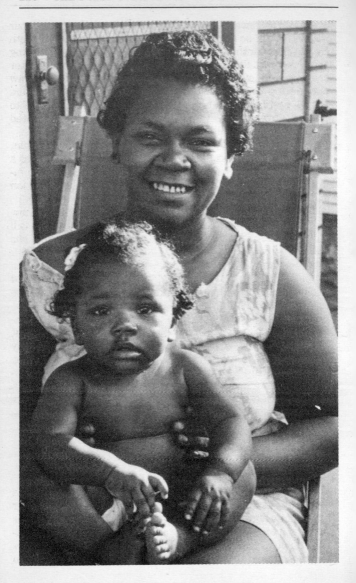

After the lower central incisors appear, the four upper incisors erupt so that the average baby has four to six teeth by his first birthday. The lower first molars, the grinding teeth farthest forward in the lower jaw, usually erupt after twelve months. A child's first teeth help to shape his jaw and determine the size of his mouth. They are space savers for his permanent teeth and should be well taken care of to prevent premature loss. Unfortunately, newly erupted teeth are especially susceptible to decay.

Most babies grind their teeth as soon as they have them, usually when they are asleep or preoccupied. This makes a terrible sound and parents fear that their children are ruining their teeth. This is not true. It serves to relieve tension and is outgrown.

Thumb-sucking can push the upper front baby teeth forward and the lower front teeth backward. However, it will have no effect on the permanent teeth if the child has stopped sucking his thumb by the time he is six years old. Stopping thumb-sucking early will cause the baby teeth to move back into place within a few months. A pacifier should not be substituted for thumb-sucking, because it will have the same effect of pushing the teeth out of line.

All medical, dental, and public-health associations recommend the addition of fluoride to drinking water unless it occurs naturally. It has been found that less tooth decay occurs where fluoride is naturally present in the water. Fluoride is added to many public water systems now as a preventive measure. A baby born to a mother who drank fluoridated water while pregnant will have 40 percent fewer cavities than a fetus not exposed to water containing fluoride.

Dental Care

Begin cleaning your baby's teeth and gums as soon as his first tooth erupts. Use a wet washcloth or a gauze pad, or a baby toothbrush with very soft bristles. If your child is taking a fluoride supplement, on your doctor's recommendation, do not dilute it with milk or juice. For maximum effectiveness, it is best to give it to him when his teeth are clean.

A Special Style

Since this is the first month that physical activity is really remarkable, differences in style grow more apparent. A baby will select stimulation compatible with his disposition just as he will resist coercion, and each baby will handle coercion differently from his peers. Some babies spend most of their waking hours practicing how to sit, roll over, or creep. Others lie quietly, looking at and listening to things. There is just no prescribed learning order or speed.

Some infants become interested in their hands only after they have mastered large movements like sitting and standing. A few master both areas—small muscles and large movements—simultaneously. Some first learn to control the small muscles of their bodies—signaled by interest in their

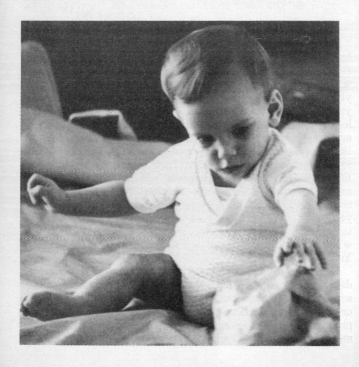

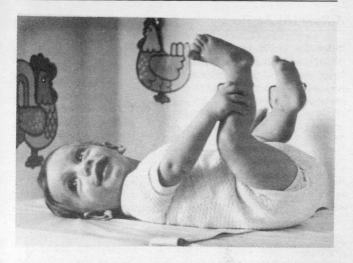

hands—and then master large movements. They may flop to one side or the other of their chairs and remain immobile when placed on their tummies. Your baby may be limp as you lift him. He may not even try to hold up his head. When you seat him on the floor his legs may poke out determinedly left and right instead of forming a triangular brace for balance. He may slump forward until his chin almost grazes the rug. If you try pulling him to stand, his legs and trunk sag. If you hold him up under the arms, he leans over your hands, sags, or sticks his legs straight out at a 90-degree angle to his trunk. This movement, which requires just as much energy as standing, may cue you to something that your baby is trying to tell you. He simply will not be pushed to perform until he's ready to do things himself, despite what the neighbors say or what *their* children are doing. You might take the tip.

Keeping your cool about your baby's more sedate motor development may be difficult, especially because of comparisons to other babies' feats. There is no reason to be alarmed or to push him. Although a complete lack of opportunity to practice things like creeping or standing may slow development, the maturing of your baby's muscles is the main antecedent of each physical ability. Bear in mind that there is no requirement that a baby sit, creep, or stand at six months. In fact, most American babies sit and creep at seven months and stand at nine or ten. Infants who respond physically to light stroking of their skin are less likely to exert muscular effort than infants who respond only to more vigorous touching. Quiet babies enjoy being tucked into bed and being dressed, even during the months of intense motor learning, and may prefer cuddly toys. Quiet infants, it has been suggested, gradually evolve greater attention spans. In school they are more able to concentrate their energies on learning.

Quieter babies also tend to be plumper than active, wiry ones, independent of food intake. According to a fascinating study at Harvard's Department of Pediatrics, thin babies moved more and ate more than average while the extremely fat ones moved and ate less. Fat babies remained fat despite unusually low calorie intake. The researchers found that unusually heavy and unusually thin babies have a smaller and larger number of active cells and, therefore, lower and higher basic metabolism than average. Basic metabolism, which is inborn, is a cause rather than a result of unusual fat proportions. The average, healthy, well-fed baby, it seems, tends to adjust his food intake to his expenditure on activity. Activity was also associated with parental characteristics. Active infants were children of sensitive, nervous, or restless parents. The less active babies had either more secure and placid parents or relatively insecure and passive parents. The children of the placid parents were more likely to increase their activity with age than those of the passive parents, who presented less stimulating environments.

The parent of an active baby should try not to worry that he sleeps less than most babies his age, or that very little food manages to get into him, or that he is not gaining enough weight. Intelligent, active, curious children, according to several studies, tend to sleep less than average. Your baby's body is geared differently than most and may be more efficient in using food and rest.

Remember, too, that during the first year, energy expended on activity peaks at six months. Your baby needs only a very few calories for growth of new tissues or weight gain. In fact, growth per se uses less than 15 percent of the total calories the baby consumes. The balance is used for daily activity.

Also, a baby simply stops gaining weight from time to time. In one study, infants who gained weight more gradually over a fifty-day period developed motor skills more quickly than infants showing rapid weight gain. Conversely, changes in a baby's body proportions and fat mass require more adjustment in the development of motor skills. In fact, physical, mental, or emotional growth proceeds in spurts, lulls, or regressions. Sometimes a baby economizes in some areas to grow or recover in others. A sick baby lacks energy for complex emotional adjustments or new mental accomplishments.

A parent of a big baby—sixteen pounds and above is heavy at this age—may establish an undesirable cycle. The baby's weight can "immobilize" him. As the baby becomes frustrated with his difficulty in moving, he may want to eat more or the parent may feed him more to keep him quiet. This is the worst thing to do, for it will establish an association between eating and relief of discomfort. It also produces excess fat cells that will become a permanent part of the body. Research indicates that an adult who has been significantly overweight since childhood can keep trim only by incessant self-denial. The extra-generous supply of greedy fat cells seems to trigger metabolic changes so that a once-fat man must restrict himself to far fewer calories to maintain a comfortable weight than a man of the same size who has never been fat.

Instead of feeding your baby more, try to encourage activity by playing vigorously with him. Peekaboo, for example, may make him bounce and "reach" with excitement. As the baby becomes more active, the fat will be used and absorbed into firmer flesh. Or let the baby find his own way to break the cycle. Keep in mind that the impact of activity on weight is at its height between four and six months. In other words, your baby's inactivity will probably be more responsible for excess weight now. Your baby's food intake, which you can pretty much control, will affect his weight more later on. Your control of his food intake plus promotion of physical activity should do the trick.

Declaration of Independence

If you are still nursing your baby, his new teeth may mean some adjustment for both of you. Of course it is accidental, but being bitten in such a sensitive place is painful and annoying. An honest reaction—startling or pushing the baby away or providing a substitute biting object (even a finger)—will help the baby learn that his behavior is unacceptable to you as much as you love him.

Bottle-feeding poses its own dilemmas. If your baby is particularly precocious, he may insist on manipulating his own bottle. Let him try it, but do continue to hold him even if he does not seem to want it at first. The most grown-up kind of baby will eventually show his appreciation of the warmth and stimulation of body contact and human exchange. A highly geared baby especially needs this to soothe him to a state in which he can absorb the warmth and gratification of feeding times. His energy and drive can push him to a kind of fierce "busyness" that lets in a very few cues from his environment.

A six-month-old may relish being started on drinking from a cup. Initially without finesse, a baby's first ventures will probably feature more chokes than swallows. But even breathing liquid up their noses will not daunt some. An infant can become so attached to his cup that he squeals or claps his hands as he sees it coming and cries if he loses it.

Even though a precocious six-month-old can probably master drinking from a cup, he should have the chance to return to his bottle whenever he seems to need it. Such regressions to more "infantile" states are necessary in the hectic pell-mell growth of the first year. Solids are something else. By this stage, your baby may also show definite likes and dislikes. Most babies, for example, refuse spinach but adore fruits. Many dislike the taste of plain meat. If yours does, you can mix the meat with a vegetable. Most babies can handle it this way. Meat is just too valuable to omit. Its iron and protein are increasingly important as your infant grows and becomes more active.

Mealtimes, you will find, are also a lot messier. The baby is more distractible and active. Feeding him in his bounce chair is worth a try. The tray holds his spoon and cup. Your six-month-old is sloppy and, believe it or not, a rain slicker may be very useful garb for his feedings. A baby can and will refuse to swallow a bite just to tease his mother, grab the spoon from her hand, sling food around the room, blow bubbles with the carrots, and spray the wall with blown-out spinach.

One reason for chaotic feedings is your baby's increased dexterity. He is ready and willing to use his hands. Like most early learning, the baby's first attempts to secure things, edible and otherwise, are terribly rigid. Even a baby's attentiveness at this time is limited by a kind of inflexibility. Researchers at Harvard's Center for Cognitive Studies found that babies around five months of age could not accommodate presentations of alternating objects that appeared less than six seconds apart. They showed a kind of overload reaction, looked puzzled, averted their heads, cried, and sometimes laughed.

To reach, a six-month-old concentrates totally on the task at hand and opens his eyes and hands *wide*. His fingers are stiffly and fully extended, and his trunk and head must be more or less aligned. The reach itself may be with both arms. It looks more like a locked pounce than a smooth act. By the end of the year, though, he will be quite dexterous.

Because of the beginning control of his small muscles, a baby this age may be interested in manipulating bits of food on his tray, closing his palm around them and taking them to his face. At this point he may try to smear the mangled residue into his mouth. Some babies are less awkward than this. A dexterous six-month-old may postpone and savor the coming pleasure of a teething biscuit for many minutes, depending on his style, then bring it to his lips and lick it all over before chewing on it. Once finished, he may lick his fingers delicately. Giving the baby teething biscuits or little pieces of toast or banana to handle while you feed him his solids will keep him happy and occupied and will encourage his important practice of manipulation.

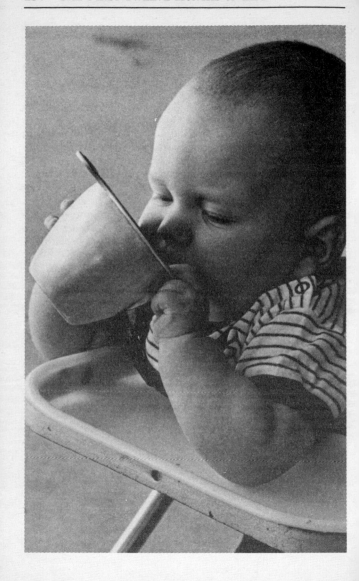

Self-Feeding

How you handle the beginning attempts at self-feeding is very important. When your baby begins grabbing at the spoon, give him one of his own to experiment with as you continue to feed him. In fact, the more your baby is permitted to help at mealtime, the faster he will learn to eat on his own. Giving him finger foods he can handle, and ignoring his sloppiness, will contribute to the ease with which he will make the transition to complete self-feeding. If a baby is never allowed to feed himself with his fingers, he will be less likely to have the ambition to try the spoon later.

At about six months, a baby is able to hold his own zwieback, and how he progresses from this stage depends largely upon your attitude. Babies make an unbelievable mess with a zwieback, which increases as they move through the finger-food stage and attempt to develop skill with a spoon.

Select nutritional foods that your baby is capable of eating. There are lots of foods from the family menu that your baby can probably handle and enjoy experimenting with. The suggestions below are to be offered in minute quantities in the beginning: dry cereal, mashed potato, almost any fruit (except strawberries), cooked rice, crumbled broiled hamburger, spaghetti, noodles and other pasta, cooked carrot pieces, bits of cooked string beans, bits of cheese, bits of French toast, teething biscuits, graham crackers, and shortbread cookies.

Of course, if your baby consistently gags, chokes, or throws up any of the finger foods, discontinue the culprit for a few weeks and talk to your pediatrician. Should you be seriously concerned about your baby's nutrition, a vitamin preparation may be suggested by your pediatrician.

"Be calm and patient" is a basic rule for every mealtime. Parents who pace feedings to their babies' wishes, respond promptly to their signals of hunger, and allow them to participate in their feedings most often experience mutually satisfying relations with their children.

Games Babies Play

Mealtimes are also the arena for games. A six-month-old loves to clown and make faces. Since meals are key socializing events, a six-month-old is very likely to try out his glad bag of facial tricks with a favorite brother or sister. Since he's not too versatile, the game will inevitably deteriorate into blowing bubbles with his milk and spitting food bits. If you can occasionally tolerate the mess, your baby will learn more than you can calculate. The games babies play help them learn the essentials of getting about in this world.

The tot who stretches his arm to his lead level when his father asks "How big are you?" is approaching the vast field of spatial relationships. The eight-month-old who plumps a block into a jar is delving into the notions of container and contained, empty and full, in and out. The ten-month-old who cruises to the stove and pokes it tentatively is ready to learn about heat and cold. The six-month-old whose favorite toy is a piece of paper that he can touch, look at, turn, rattle, crackle, change its shape by bending or rolling, and finally take to his mouth and savor is experimenting with the properties of objects.

Peekaboo, a game that appears about the beginning of the fifth month, is in the same class. Its first version involves the parent hiding his face with his hands, then removing them, much to the baby's delight. The baby soon learns to cover his own face. The game is so instinctive that a healthy infant may draw other relatives into the fun. Sibs play the game more vigorously, leap from behind chairs, roar and yell. The baby is enchanted with either variant and even stops crying to play them. Within weeks of its appearance, the baby himself will invent variations. He draws a diaper over his face, chuckles, and kicks his feet playfully after calling his parents. They ask, "Where is baby?" He squeals with delight and keeps the diaper on. If they remain quiet too long, the baby may vocalize and kick again, then remove the diaper from a startled little face to smile, reassured by their presence. Peekaboo may be a first token of humor. Baby has played a trick on someone and has clearly decided beforehand that he in fact intended to play one.

The game also means the baby has a memory of someone he loves, and his or her image is fixed enough in his mind and secure enough in his feelings for him to try a short separation under his control. It also means that he has a sense of mother's permanence, as well as that of objects, and even anticipates the joy of recalling her.

A bit later, the baby will assay separations in other ways. The come-and-get-me game requires a pursuing parent and a scrambling baby. The game should not be curtailed too quickly lest you end up with a furious infant. Several runs before the abduction of the infant to a meal or a diaper change will promote a more resigned capitulation. At about the same age, a baby may begin to look over the edge of his chair at objects that he has dropped to the floor. This is the pick-up-the-things-I-drop game. He will vary this during feeding times by dropping his spoon and cup overboard as he avoids the spoon you proffer. When all droppable items are gone, he will probably cry for parent or sibs to retrieve them.

As with peekaboo, this game demonstrates that the baby is beginning to have a concept of himself. He is separate from other people and from objects and can influence them through actions *he* has selected. In a more general sense, his initiation of the game relates to a growing capacity to formulate a goal and take the necessary actions to attain it. Intent matched with a plan is nothing short of intelligent behavior.

Of course, brothers and sisters can expand this repertoire endlessly. Together they can romp around the house. Despite the risks of accidentally being stepped on or spilled from a chair, this play is very valuable. As your baby cooperates with his sibs, he develops mentally and socially. He has opportunities to touch, watch, imitate, and listen that he would otherwise never have. He learns he must sometimes "play" a role to hold someone's attention. A brother or sister for the baby is an advantage to you, too. He may violently refuse your feeding but sit quietly for a bowl of cereal or even an entire meal from his sister. On a particularly bad day, you have one more resource on which to rely.

Play with brothers or sisters is so rewarding that a baby

will gladly overcome pain, fear, or reprimands to keep them near. A baby is a resilient little creature, and almost nothing a brother or sister can do will frighten him. Sibs will distract your baby from his growing pains, fill in your temporary absences, and actually assist in your caring for him. They can stimulate a quiet baby or slow a hyperactive one with pastimes such as "reading" that he would otherwise not tolerate except for his love of them. Because of them, an inner-directed baby will grow interested in something besides his own activity. Play with toys and things that require him to utilize his hands, and sharing play might otherwise be longer and harder in coming. Hopefully, you will agree that this play means so much to your baby and other children in learning to build relationships and growing to love each other that you will carefully monitor it, interfere when necessary but not stop it because of some relatively minor risks.

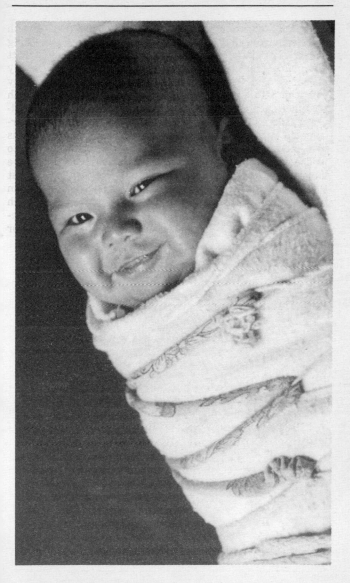

Interactive Games for Parents and Baby

Mothers and fathers everywhere have invented tickling games that are remarkably similar in vastly different cultures. In these games, the parent uses two fingers to simulate the walking of a mouse, rabbit, or spider up the baby's body from his toes, up his arm from his hand, or from his wrist to his neck. The parent surprises the baby by tickling him at "tickle spots" under the arm or chin or behind the ears. An accompanying verse might be:

> Creepie mousie, creepie mousie,
> In the barn and over the housie,
> And in the baby's kitty housie.

Below are some interactive games you will be able to play with your baby by the time he is eight or nine months old, or perhaps sooner.
English verse:

> Round and round the garden like a teddy bear,
> One step, two step, and tickly under there.

Action: Parent walks two fingers around in the baby's palm and then tickles him at the elbow and the upper arm. At "and tickly under there," the baby is tickled under his arm.
American verse:

> Hickory, dickory, dock!
> The mouse ran up the clock.
> The clock struck one, and down he run.
> Hickory, dickory, dock!

Action: The parent walks fingers up and down the baby from feet to neck and from neck to feet.
English verse:

> Ride a cock horse to Banbury Cross,
> To see a fine lady upon a white horse;
> With rings on her fingers and bells on her toes,
> She shall have music wherever she goes.

(continued)

In playing "Ride a Cock Horse," the parent crosses one knee over the other and perches his or her baby on the free foot. The baby's hands are held as the parent moves the free leg up and down rhythmically while singing.

Your baby's eyes will be glued to your face. He will smile at the end of the game and let you know by jiggling himself up and down that he wants you to do it again. Sing, and do the game again. It's great fun for both of you.

Some tactile games emphasize fingers and toes. They often include a sensational tickling finish. In "This Little Pig Went to Market," for instance, the parent takes each toe in turn, wriggling each gently while reciting what each piggy does:

> This little pig went to market;
> This little pig stayed home;
> This little pig had roast beef;
> This little pig had none;
> And this little pig cried, "Wee, wee, wee!"
> All the way home.

At "wee, wee, wee," the parent tickles the baby on the tummy or under the chin. In China, the baby's toes are cows:

> This little cow eats grass,
> This little cow eats hay,
> This little cow drinks water,
> This little cow runs away.
> This little cow does nothing
> But lie down all day.

There are several ways to induce crescendoes in order to produce frolic and laughter in babies. The parent kisses the baby on the hand, on the wrist, on the elbow, on the arm, and finally on the cheek, to the accompaniment of chuckles and laughter.

(continued)

"The Beehive" rhyme highlights the fingers:

Here is the beehive. Where are the bees? [Hold hand in
a fist.]
Hidden away where nobody sees.
Soon they come creeping out of the hive [Relax fist.]
One! two! three! four! five! [Extend thumb, index,
second, ring, and small fingers.]
As the baby grows increasingly aware of his body parts
and his distinctiveness from other people, he will
appreciate the separateness of his fingers and toes.
The time for vigorous rocking games is when your baby is
able to sit propped in a chair for long periods of time.
Chances are your baby will be dissatisfied with just the
gentle rocking of lullabies or cars that used to almost
mesmerize him. Father's bouncing him on his foot
becomes far more entrancing.
American verse:

Chop, chop to Boston,
Chop, chop to Lynn.
Careful when you get there,
You don't fall IN!

Action: The father bounces the baby on his knees and
then lets the baby fall in between his legs as he carefully
supports the baby's upper back, neck, and head.

Naming games, involving the baby's nose, toes, feet,
hands, and mouth, emphasize body parts, as well as the
concept of self. Cues for such games usually come from
the baby. As part of exploring and comparing himself to
his world and the people in it, your baby will poke at his
ears, nose, mouth, and eyes (yours, too), and may even
compare the feel of your features with his. If you suck his
exploring finger, he may try sucking it again himself, then
offer it to you for a resampling.

A favorite nursery rhyme that contrasts the size of the
parent's and the baby's hands also shows their similarity
in shape:

(continued)

> Pat-a-cake, pat-a-cake,
> Baker man!
> Bake me a cake,
> As fast as you can.
> Pat it, and prick it,
> And mark it with B.
> Put it in the oven
> For Baby and me!
>
> Action: The parent takes the baby's hands and claps them together. In time, the baby will clap his hands against those of his parent.
>
> As interactive games bring pleasure to parents and baby, they also enhance the baby's sense of well-being and security and add to his mental development and boundless feeling of self-esteem.

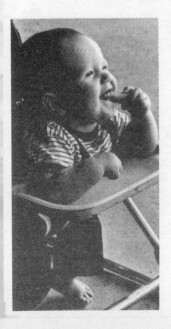
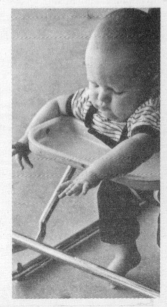

THE SIXTH MONTH

Motor Development	Language
### *Gross Motor*	### *Vocalizing*

Gross Motor

Moro reflex; startling when pillow or side of crib is struck; the arms and legs flex to body. Terminates between six and nine months. Swimming reflex disappears.

Turns head freely.

Voluntary creeping appears. Crawling reflex disappears and voluntary crawling begins.

On back, grasps foot in play.

On tummy, lifts and extends legs high. Turns, twists in all directions. Rolls from back to stomach. May get up on hands and knees in crouch, hurtle forward or backward by flinging limbs out. Creeps—propels self on tummy with legs, steers with arms, goes backward or forward.

Stands with substantial support.

Sitting

Sits with slight support; balances well. Can lean forward or to side. Sits in chair, grasps dangling object. Bounces.

Sits alone momentarily. May sit unsupported up to half an hour. May need to slump forward on hands to balance.

May bend self to near-sitting position on side while rolling from back.

Vocalizing

Vowels begin to be interspersed with more consonants (*f, v, th, s, sh, z, sz, m, n,* commonly). Varies volume, pitch, rate of utterance.

All vocalizations still differ from mature language, but more control of sounds.

Babbles and becomes active during exciting sounds. Babbles back most to female voices.

Vocalizes pleasure and displeasure; grunts, growls or complains; coos, gurgles with pleasure; squeals with excitement; giggles, belly-laughs.

Vocalizes at mirror image.

Responding

Reacts to differences in intonations and inflections.

Responds to sounds of words (not to their meaning).

Mental	Social

Mental

Sensory Response

Turns head to human sounds or sounds of objects out of sight. Coos or hums or stops crying on hearing music. Reacts to changes in volume.

Hand preference emerges. Mouths objects.

Attention Span

Alert two hours at a stretch. Visually alert close to 50 percent of daylight hours.

Eye-Hand Coordination

Reaches persistently, quickly, and without jerks for anything he sees. Usually looks at anything he reaches for, but may close eyes. Picks up block deftly and directly. Likes to look at objects upside down and to create changes in perspective. Inspects objects at length. Lifts cup by handle. Pulls paper away. Shows interest in containers. Lifts inverted containers. Explores objects by shaking, hitting, dropping, throwing. Loses sight of object and searches for it (object permanence).

Reaches to grab and secure dropped object.

As a result of sitting posture, curiosity and exploration are reaching a new high, which will be satisfied only when infant begins to crawl on his own.

Social

Personal

Smiles at mirror image. Differentiates self from mirror image.

Alternates hand with object in mouth; alternates hands to hold objects—aware of separate parts of self, self versus world. Tries to imitate facial expression. Turns when he hears name.

Interaction

Is more discriminating about people he responds to. Beginning of stranger anxiety; reacting with hesitation and fear to people other than immediate family members.

Distinguishes adults from children. Smiles at, reaches out to pat strange children. Calls parents for help.

Cultural Self-Help/Routines

Begins to show interest in finger-feeding self. Develops strong taste preferences. May want to manipulate own bottle. May start manipulating cup.

Sleeps through night. Sleeps about half of 24-hour period.

Play and Playthings

Prefers play with people, especially interacting games: peekaboo, come-and-get-me, go-and-fetch.

(continued)

Motor Development	Language
Fine Motor Holds bottle. Rotates wrist. Turns, manipulates objects. Reaches with one arm. Is fascinated with very small particles: bread crumbs, pebbles, marbles, etc. (under supervision, of course).	

Please do not regard this chart as a rigid timetable. Babies are unpredictable. Some perform an activity earlier or later than the chart indicates.

Mental	Social

Memory

Grasps with fingers, examines object, and makes "motor copies" in brain.

Staring behavior, the result of visual acumen. Using hands as a tool to reach and explore nearby objects enables baby to build a base of intelligence.

Body and Object Awareness

Attends to another's scribbling.

Senses the relationship between hands and objects they manipulate.

Discriminating and Associating

Transfers object from one hand to the other. Holds one block, reaches for a second. Regards third block immediately.

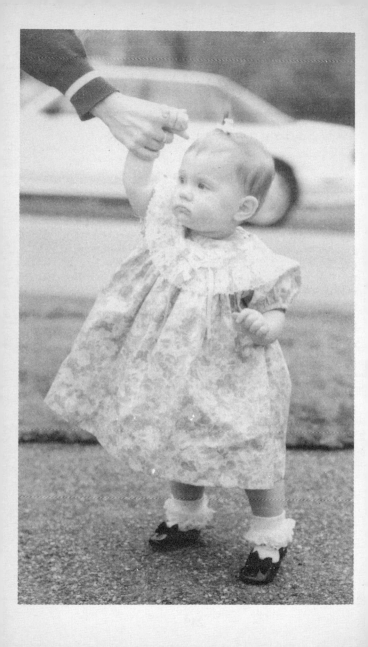

The Seventh Month

PERPETUAL MOTION

During the second half of this first year of life, your baby's overall body proportions will change rapidly, and he will move from relative immobility to the basic skills that will enable him to get about in his world. For most babies, the seventh month is one big gush of motor development. While your baby has been sitting supported for several months, he can sit all by himself now for many minutes and can be carried comfortably on your hip. The use of his arms and hands, at last free from supporting him, give him a new lease on life, and the greater agility of his trunk lets him begin to wheel around and lean over to pick up objects, which he deliberately drops just to practice his new picking-up skill. He can turn himself over halfway from his stomach and push with his arms on one side to a sitting position. Some will try one side, drop back to the ground and try the other, as if delighting in full exploration of each before settling on one.

The baby's creeping improves visibly and he can count on going forward all of the time. He may start to practice some variations on this theme. Above all, he is beginning to experiment with standing. In the next few months, he will convert his world from a sitting-down to a standing-up one. Of course, the baby's budding ability to get about and his growing activity have far-reaching implications for him and for his family.

Many babies begin to practice crawling this month, the first really effective way to get about. Crawling is a difficult art, according to Dr. Myrtle McGraw, a developmental psychologist who has studied infant physical development for almost forty years. She writes that "nowhere is the struggle between higher and lower brain centers for the control of behavior more clear than in the development of crawling." The higher brain, or cortex, does not take over the movement of all muscle groups in this activity at the same time. It begins with the shoulders and arms and eventually gets to the legs. So for a while at the beginning of cortex functioning, your baby will pull and tug with his arms trying to move himself forward, while the legs hang behind like a dead weight. Or he may push up on his hands, straighten his arms, and twist from one side to the other. Eventually he might flex his legs and hop on his knees. Some babies will get up on palms and knees, rock back and forth, or hurtle forward before really shoving off properly.

Eventually your baby may push up on his legs and "practice" this new accomplishment for hours on end.

For a couple of weeks or so, he may simply teeter on four small stilts. Then he may apply information about locomo-

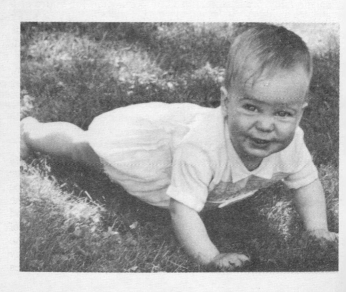

tion that he gained from creeping and gingerly inch a stiffened leg out and move a little. The first participation of the legs is only halfhearted. One leg goes this way, and one that. An arm swings out twice before a leg can be persuaded to move; and sometimes the baby loses his usual control of shoulders and arms and falls flat on his face. A few more tries and he learns that a hitch with a foot can be followed by a hitch with one arm. The two supports balance better, and he begins to get the leg and arm on one side to work with each other. He plops on his nose many times more before he realizes that he also has to fetch the opposite leg and arm. Ultimately, the body and four limbs begin to work together as a precision team. Dr. Brazelton suggests that there may be inborn corrections between motor acts that feel "right" when made by chance and integrated. These connections send a rewarding signal to the baby's brain, which allows the baby to identify and preempt that piece of experimentation for the next try.

Dr. McGraw was among the first to detail this relentless practice of a motor task until it is thoroughly mastered. Just as the baby practices his ground locomotion for hours at a stretch, so he practices standing. One day you may be lucky enough to witness your baby's first efforts. His playpen is often the easiest place to start. It offers lots of easy handgrips. Or he may maneuver over to a large piece of furniture, like the couch or a buffet, gather his knees under him, pull with his arms and push with his legs. Finally, he has gotten *himself* to stand.

Variations on a Theme

No infant, however, need subscribe to such rituals. Babies differ in the order and speed with which they learn motor skills. A small apartment, unlike a large house, may reduce a baby's incentive to keep up with his mother because he can see and hear her from any room. Some babies will stand between creeping and crawling. This curious interlocking of developmental steps is not uncommon. Some babies become frightened by their sudden ability to stand. As if struck by the need for more ground practice, they plump themselves down again to drill an alternative pattern on hands and knees. After they absorb it, they stand again several weeks later, reassured enough to attack the important step of upright locomotion. Because of this kind of unevenness in growth—the lags and lulls that every baby experiences—you should know when not to drive your baby in a given direction, as well as when to stimulate and encourage the expansion of some performance.

For a very active baby, sitting alone may be old hat at this point, and creeping, passé. On the other hand, a quiet baby may just be learning to inch along by seven months and won't even begin to crawl until the tenth. While creeping usually precedes crawling by several months, your baby's crawling may follow in a month's time. An active baby may navigate by half rolling, half pushing at five months; move with speed at six months; and crawl this month, compared to the "average" baby, who creeps at six months and crawls efficiently at eight.

Babies also differ in the type of locomotive skills they favor. Dr. McGraw writes of the many fascinating styles with which babies first learn to get about, styles that often seem to reflect the baby's character. One style, a sitting position in which the baby uses one arm for pulling and one leg for pushing, frees a baby's eyes and ears for every nuance in the environment. This sitting posture may be associated with a baby who is extra sensitive to sights and sounds. It also leaves him in a better position to retrieve toys and to continue playing with them once he arrives at his destination.

An inactive infant may already be adding other forms of locomotion, ground and upright, to his inventory. He sits and bounces across the floor on his buttocks, a method that replaces creeping for some babies.

A very active baby may also be able to move about standing up, by lunging and grabbing one piece of furniture after another. Although his balance is shaky and he may fall forward repeatedly, his bravado will probably remain unscathed as he gradually refines his judgments.

A quiet baby may quite legitimately be doing very different things. During this month his activity may spurt. He is much more cooperative in sitting when a parent helps him, and he can sit alone by hunching forward and supporting himself on both arms. If your baby is doing this about now, don't leave him this way too long or he will tire the sparse musculature of his lower back. In his own leisurely manner, he will also begin to move. On his back he can mosey along by hoisting his buttocks and pushing with his feet. Since this works him toward new places, he gains incentive to move, not because he enjoys movement in itself as some babies do, but because it brings a change of scene and new visual delights. If he is intrigued with sound as well as sight, he will appreciate the splatting noise of his buttocks as he flops along. He, too, practices for long hours in his own fashion.

To encourage a quiet baby to locomote on his stomach, place a favorite toy just out of reach. As soon as he realizes you won't get it for him, he may hump grudgingly toward it. Selective doses of frustration often give an important and sometimes necessary push toward learning. Make sure the toy itself is attractive. If your baby is relatively indifferent toward motor performance, the strategy may otherwise fail.

This same baby may be quite precocious in the use of his hands. He can use this as an outlet as much as another baby uses large motor achievements. In comparison to a baby who is precocious in both large and small muscular achievement, your baby may be very conservative in sitting, moving, and standing but still excel in manipulative skill. He may amuse himself on his stomach for thirty minutes, fingering a string of small beads of different shapes and textures. He loves to play with a cluster of keys, handling, rattling, and mouthing each. He can reach, poke at, and pick up even a minute puff of dust in a thumb and forefinger.

If your baby can sit unsupported on the floor, pick up a cup with one hand, and carry it to his mouth using both hands, then he is precocious indeed. Usually, a seven-month-old can handle only much larger objects. He is not nearly as sophisticated about shape, texture, or his own grasping style. Now that his thumb fully apposes his fingers, he can grasp blocks or toys comfortably. Joyously he bangs together toys held in each hand or hits one, then the other against the floor or wall, much like his mirrored, alternating arm and leg activity as a newborn. At this stage, play in front of a mirror helps your baby sort the merits of one side against the other—a part of finding out about his world. Although some babies start to prefer the right to the left side of their body as early as three or four months, most infants use both hands equally all through the first year. Holding a block in each hand simultaneously previews another new and exciting accomplishment, the use of both hands instead of only one or the other.

Experimentation with his hands is so exciting that a seven-month-old usually appears with something in one or the other. He creeps around a room dangling a toy, and sometimes keeps both hands occupied. Even standing, he hangs onto a support with one hand while manipulating a toy with the other.

Exploring the World

With his increased dexterity, mobility, and curiosity, your baby will begin to explore everything as he pulls himself around the house. That is one reason babyproofing your house is so important. Anything to do with electricity should be protected *and* designated as a definite no. Plastic covers should fill up electrical outlets. If the baby's finger is wet or if he pokes his tongue into an outlet, he can burn himself badly. And an electric burn does not heal without scarring. You must also stay close to the baby now on his home-world tours, even though an enjoyable companion will only spur him on to further adventures.

As part of exploring and comparing himself to his world and the people in it, the baby may poke at your ears, nose, mouth, and eyes, as well as his own, and even compare the feel of your features with his. If you suck his exploring finger, he may try sucking it again himself, then offer it for a resampling.

As your baby investigates, he may poke at every part of his body. He has already discovered his ears, nose, and mouth, and now as he begins to sit and bend forward, he can also see the lower part of his body. But his only real

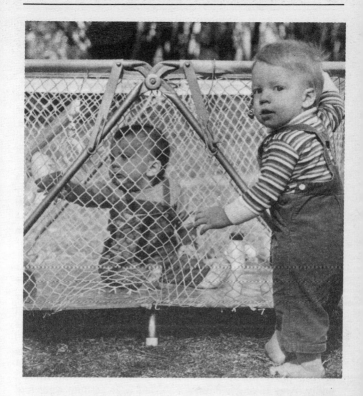

opportunity to find out about his genitals is when he is un-diapered. A baby boy may play with and pull his penis until he has an erection. A girl may poke at her vagina.

The pleasure generated when an infant first finds his genitals clearly indicates their greater sensitivity in comparison to their body parts. American practice intensifies the baby's curiosity and pleasure and heightens sensitivity. Our puritan heritage makes us uncomfortable with our bodies and we keep this area hidden and out of reach. Diapers protect the genitals so well that the skin is conditioned to stimulation only with elimination. Other body parts are more exposed to air, temperature changes, pressure, and touch.

Then, too, when a baby starts investigating, somebody grabs the deviant hand, distracts him, or covers the area. Reaction varies from embarrassment and moral indignation to real concern, offense, and shock, particularly among adults of the older generation. So the baby may grow especially fascinated with this novel and provoking-to-parent region. Sometimes we justify our behavior by insisting that unless we curtail normal handling, the child will damage himself. Any competent physician can assure you that this is not so. The baby's discovery and exploration of his genitals is normal and important now and at all ages, and most babies go through it. Institutional babies are often "stuck" in it because they have nothing more pleasurable or interesting to do. But an infant with emotionally healthy parents and a stimulating environment almost never is.

The baby also goes through some emotional adjustments to his improved mobility. He is often more interested in being included in social interaction, more tense, and more dependent on mother. In his sitting-up world, the baby was willing to sit and watch, smile when his sibs smiled, and gurgle when they laughed. But now he needs to be an active participant. When his "recognize me please" need is unanswered, he either creeps into the middle of whatever they are doing or creeps to find you.

The tension before big developmental steps, like sitting and moving about, may show itself in irritability or chewing fingers and thumbs. Some babies actually look vacant and roll or bang their heads so much that their hair wears away until their tension is released in real action. Then these disturbing behaviors taper off except when the baby is tired or hungry, when he suddenly reverts to them. When life is again consistently gratifying, they will disappear as your baby, fancy free, whips through the house—his territory at last.

The baby's new freedom, because of his improved locomoting skill, also exposes him suddenly to increased stimulation from all angles before he has had the chance to adapt to it. His unreadiness, plus the sometimes frightening information he gets in his broadened sphere, make him more dependent and more fearful of separations from you.

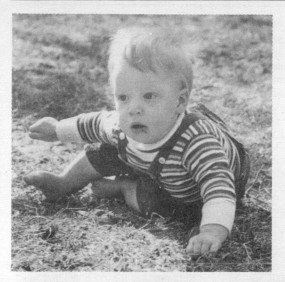

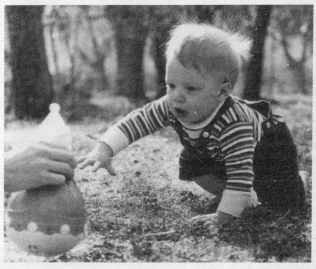

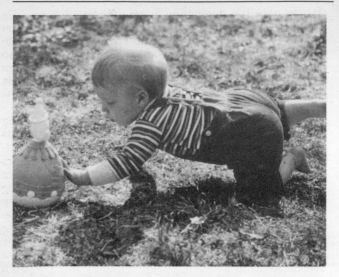

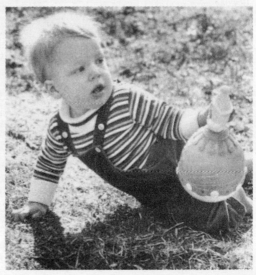

Heightening this fearfulness is his affection for you. He wants food, attention, stimulation, and approval from you even when others are available to offer them to him. He keeps close to you with a more or less primitive mental map in which you move more or less predictably. He is also more aware of your ability to move (and that means away from him) because he knows through his own experience what moving is all about.

As he performs the motor arts of standing and crawling himself, he becomes aware of their dimensions. As he stands tottering for the first time and has to be helped down, self-conscious and frightened, he becomes aware of the dangers of falling and his own inability to modify his position. Once thoroughly delighted in being pulled to stand by a loving sister, he may now steadfastly refuse to be stood up by anyone but his parents, correctly aware that their competence and judgment are greater than his. His frightening awareness that he and you can get away from each other precedes real mastery in getting away, and creates some indecision about improving this terrifying skill. The truth is that you are still much better at getting away from the baby than he is at keeping up with you.

Besides that, he is still very inept and new at his explorations and play, which are admittedly great fun. Perhaps he senses he has little discrimination about the dangers he is dimly aware of and desperately needs your help to retrieve him from the difficulties he is surely going to work himself into. As long as he sees you, he can play contentedly. You may notice that when you leave a room, he cries and tries to follow, and he no longer likes staying in his playpen while you work in another room. Although you may need to keep him in his pen, at least try to help his new dependence. When you leave, turn to tell him you'll return, and call to him periodically from the distance. The vocal contact will be some comfort, and he'll probably call you to check on your location every once in a while. Although sometimes content with this exchange, he may aim himself in your direction, facing the door you might enter or the direction of your voice, or work himself into a frenzy just to get you back so he can cling a little. Don't worry. His drive for independence, plus your reassurance and consistent presence, will press him through his temporary impasse. Attachment to a person or belief is usually most intense just after it is realized, so the baby is most vulnerable now to any brand of separation from you. Remember, too, that only babies who have good relationships with their parents are uncomfortable with separations. Babies whose parents make little difference one way or the other react less because they have learned to cope alone and too soon.

Undercover Work

Although the baby again seems to be devoting all his energy to developing his physical skills, he is also working on his mental abilities. His associations are becoming more and more keen. When he hears the front door open and close at night, he sings out to greet his father. Most of it is sheer babble, but somewhere in that stream is something like "dada." He knows that sounds of the refrigerator door mean food, and grunts in anticipation of his own feeding. As his sister imitates him by sucking her own fingers, his laughter demonstrates he already visually associates her act with his. In "reading" with a brother who "meows" for the cats and "bow-wows" for the dogs in a picture book, he crows—without prompting—at a picture of a baby as if he recognizes it and associates the baby with himself and his own sounds. He has also learned behavior immediately appropriate to his "reading." He discerns that his brother makes a sound for a picture, and does the same thing—correctly. Older women seem fine at first because he connects them with grandmother, but as soon as he takes a good look and hears the voice (corroborating evidence), he bristles with fear and disappointment. He is also becoming aware of size differences and able to sort them. Give your baby blocks of different sizes to play with and watch what he does. If he holds them out in front of him, looks from one to the other, and places them in front of him, then he is really comparing them. As if to digest their size difference, he picks them up again with different hands, mouths each, and puts them down again—in reverse order. Such comparing can occur as early as six months, but is more usual now.

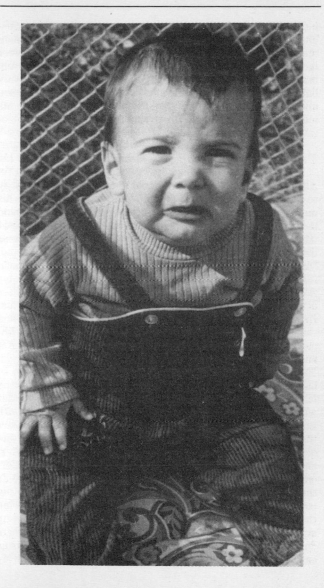

He is developing a sense of humor, which often starts with humorous, playful associations with a game or in response to a surprise situation with an adult or child. For example, if you join in your baby's singing to himself, he may stop, smile, and resume humming. He may giggle and even bounce in time with you. Sometimes a segment of the original fun situation may trigger remembrance of all of it and elicit his first response. Dr. Brazelton describes such a situation. You drop something and say "damn," and the baby laughs at the suddenness of the word and at your awkward posture as you pick it up. The association is made. You pull a laugh with a swear word every time as the baby identifies the words, sounds, and emotional overtones. Your baby, incidentally, also reinforces you. A repeated response—the baby's laughter—shows not only a general ability to remember but also the ability to remember segments representative of whole situations. This ability is precocious at seven months but quite possible.

Language Expansion

The babbling of the seven-month-old becomes enriched by two-syllable "words" that are at first linked repetitions of his early cooing sounds, e.g., "ala," "anna," "oogoo," "lala," and "looloo." Later on these repetitions come into play with such "words" as "mimi," "ippi," et cetera.

Bits and Pieces

As part of his increased dexterity, many a seven- or eight-month-old will begin to pick up bits of food with his thumb and first two fingers at mealtimes. Since he is still awkward, his self-feeding will be messy. If food drops into his closed fist, he will have to work arduously to extract it. His method of getting food into his mouth is to smear it in with his palm. When finished with what is often a long and laborious process, the baby may mash his leavings into the feeding tray or sweep them onto the floor in a grand gesture of satiety.

Despite his clumsiness, the baby should be encouraged in his desire to feed himself. Letting him participate in simple

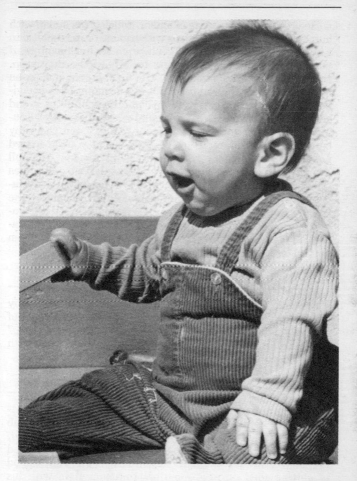

ways, like supplying finger bits or a spoon and cup for each hand is much easier for you and more informative for your baby. "Many mothers," Brazelton points out, "feel so compulsive about getting food into their babies that they miss the obvious value of the baby's exploratory behavior with it." First, the baby will learn to feed himself. He will also learn more about his environment. Looking at, handling, tasting, and smelling food is part of the same exploring that begins earlier with inedibles. A simple indication of this learning would be the baby's reluctance to finger slippery foods, such as bananas, in contrast to his crumbling cookies and breads beyond recognition. These sensuous experiences with food enhance the entire feeding exchange for your baby. If he is allowed to enjoy his food and permitted to develop his own eating habits, he also learns that the world is not a restrictive, forbidding place where assertion of his own feelings and wants only brings trouble.

In countless passive and not-so-passive ways, a baby can fight a parent who ignores his desire to participate in his own feeding. If the baby can't amuse himself, he may prolong the meal interminably. He may start to tease you by throwing bits of food around, spitting, sputtering, or delicately oozing out food after slowly and scientifically inspecting and turning it in his mouth. He may laugh joyously at his own antics, mouth full, of course. Or he may fling his head, clench his mouth, or grab for the spoon he wants to manipulate. Chewing and swallowing unwieldy lumps that he feeds himself and refusal of your smaller, more manageable ones signal the greater incentive of independent action.

Many foods can be gummed up in the baby's mouth or swallowed whole if they are diced into tiny pieces. These should be given to him in small quantities at a time so he won't stuff himself and choke.

It is still too early for a spoon and a fork. Such dexterity comes at about sixteen months. By the time he can stand and walk, a baby can feed himself entirely with finger foods, manipulate bits amazingly well, and drink from his cup with help. Right now, the baby can handle a cup awkwardly. In the first week or so of cup use, a seven-month-old has no appreciation of how to keep the rim of his cup at an angle compatible with the horizontal level of the milk, juice, or water inside. In respect for his rigid handling, try filling the cup only slightly. At fourteen months, the baby will be able to match the cup to water level with four of five corrective movements of the hands, wrists, and elbows as he lifts it to his mouth. By twenty-seven months, these distinct corrections are all gone, and the hand-wrist-arm system fluidly and smoothly maintains the levels of rim and liquid on the way to the mouth.

Feeding Problems

A mother who pressures her baby to eat can cause real feeding problems. Teasing or tricking the baby to accept the food you offer, or startling him so that you can shove food in when he drops his jaw in astonishment are the worst things you can do. They are not only cruel, they may eventually yield entrenched resistance and difficulty.

If the baby does begin to respond to your pressure with his own tension, try instead to let him gradually take over his own feeding while you busy yourself in another part of the kitchen. It will get your tension out of the situation until you cool it and let the baby handle his own dilemma. If you continue to press him beyond his interest in food, the backlash will be disproportionate to any gains made. When he becomes more active, he may ruin meals by standing in his chair to show off, ignore his food, beg for pieces of yours, then throw or smash them beyond recognition. Or he may literally cruise around the edge of the table, begging like a troublesome puppy or clawing at whatever he can see. Around twelve months of age he will demonstrate his strong determination to eat what and when he chooses even more resourcefully. He will win, or be completely beaten into uneasy submission. No baby should be allowed to use meals to provoke or heighten tension in his family. If you are clear and firm about what you expect from him and uncompelled by the size of your baby's intake, your baby will learn the social value of mealtime—for you now, and for himself later, when he will have to know it.

Dr. Mary D. Ainsworth, a well-known psychologist at The Johns Hopkins University, described how mothers' styles in feeding their babies related to later behavior. Those mothers in her studies who paced the feedings to their babies' wishes, responded promptly to signals of hunger and satisfaction, and allowed their babies to participate actively in the feeding had smooth and mutually gratifying relation-

ships with them. At the end of their first year, these babies
showed healthy, undisturbed attachments to their mothers
by actively trying to regain contact with them and to maintain it by clinging and resisting release after a brief separation. Babies whose mothers were relatively insensitive and
unresponsive to them in feeding situations lacked interest
in keeping in touch with them. Or they mixed their efforts
at contact with turning, moving, looking away, or actually
pushing the mothers away. Generally, mothers who could
see things from the baby's viewpoint adopted infant-care
practices that led to harmonious interaction in feeding and
elsewhere. Babies whose mothers consistently and interest-
ingly responded to their behavior learned ways to communicate with the mother other than by hard crying. They could
also tolerate frustration better than babies whose behavior
made little or no difference in determining what happened
to them. Allowing a baby autonomy consistent with his interest and capacity seems to be part of rearing a healthy,
happy child.

Fear of Strangers

In the middle of his first year, a baby is likely to develop an
intense fear of strangers and strange places. On seeing a
new face, he will bury his head in his mother's or his father's
neck and scream loudly, causing the onlooker to feel rejected
and even guilty. Unfortunately, the onlooker can be a grandparent. This is an easy problem to overcome. Left alone to
adjust, the baby will eventually seek out the stranger, first
with his eyes and then with an actual overture of friendship.

Head Banging, Head Rolling, and Jouncing

Toward the second half of the first year, a baby sometimes
takes to banging his head hard and rhythmically against the
crib or rolling it from side to side, or he may get on his
hands and knees and jounce against his heels in a steady
rhythm. Head banging is especially disturbing and frightening to parents. They are afraid their baby will hurt himself,

and sometimes even imagine that he is lacking in intelligence. Even when they are reassured that this banging will not injure his brain and that it is not a sign of any kind of mental abnormality, it is nerve-racking for them to listen to the constant thudding.

Why do babies do this? No one seems to know for sure. Apparently jouncing and head banging occur mostly when a baby is going to sleep or is partially awake. Many babies do not go directly to sleep. They first seem to go through a short period of tenseness. Head banging, head rolling, and jouncing, as well as thumb-sucking or clutching a favorite toy or blanket, may be the baby's way of ameliorating his tension.

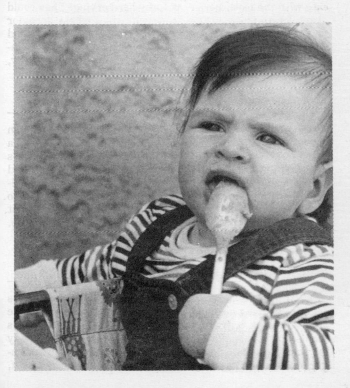

It is suggested that such a baby may need more cuddling than he is getting. Pediatricians advise against scolding the baby or trying to restrain him physically, because both of these measures would only make him more tense. If your baby bangs his head, you can line the crib with quilted padding so he will not bruise himself. Try padding the outside of the crib if it thumps against the wall.

It will not be long before your baby will outgrow this behavior, but he will probably get over it more readily if you can relax and take sufficient time to cuddle and enjoy him. It sometimes is helpful to synchronize a metronome to the tempo of the child's banging and place it near the crib, or you might try a radio tuned to a classical-music station. Sometimes a warm bath just before bedtime will have the effect of relaxing your baby so that he will go right to sleep.

Sleep

As with everything else, each baby's need for sleep varies considerably. However, most babies spend less time sleeping as they approach their first-year birthday. Research indicates that although the average number of hours of sleep is about thirteen for most babies from six to twelve months of age, many babies sleep anywhere from nine to eighteen hours daily. In fact, most babies usually sleep as much as they need to.

At six or seven months, most babies fall asleep easily unless they are kept awake by hunger, pain, or illness. This changes at about nine months and thereafter, when babies may keep themselves awake deliberately, or they are unable to fall asleep due to excessive stimulation or stress around their bedtime. Also, they may want to be part of the family action for longer periods of time.

If your baby has a hard time going to sleep, do not let him cry alone, but when you go to comfort him, do not pick him up. Talk to him gently, pat him on the back, and let him know it is time for him to go to sleep. You may have to do this multiple times before he gets the message, but he will.

The combination of teething and fears may cause sleep problems at this age. Giving your baby a routine bedtime and a few minutes to calm himself after being put down for the night may lead to easier bedtimes.

Play and Playthings

The crawling baby loves to hide under tables, under bottom shelves, in closets, and in corners. He pulls at accessible drawers. He often gets stuck between a table and chair legs. There is need for "peekaboo houses," contoured surfaces with "nests" in which the crawler can cuddle up, and floor and wall "busy boxes" with programmed challenges. Try making a vari-textured carpet for your baby's playpen.

Preparing a proper environment for the crawler is the parents' responsibility, because few toymakers provide playthings for the crawling-exploring set. Also, this is the time to put safety locks on all cabinets and to move all fragile objects beyond your baby's reach.

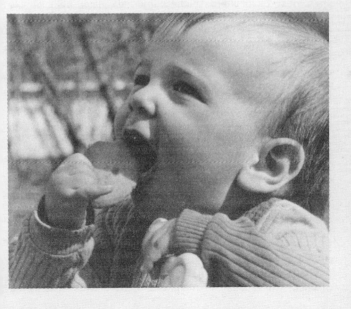

Intention and Goal-seeking Behavior

At this stage, the infant moves from being primarily a reflexive organism who responds in undifferentiated ways to his environment to being a relatively coherent organization of sensorimotor powers. He begins to demonstrate intention and goal seeking. Now his motions are no longer completely random or accidental. He pulls a knob because he knows this will cause a bell to ring. He drops something on the floor because he wants to hear the noise or make his parent come running. Your baby's actions are "lived" rather than thought about.

Manipulating the Environment

During the six- to twelve-month period, countless actions and manipulations on the environment are the way an infant gets a "picture of things." There are innumerable things that must be brought to the baby's attention that he can explore with his hands, mouth, feet, arms, and body. From a vast variety of play experiences, he gets a feeling of size, shape, texture, weight, volume, density, distance, speed, and altitude, among other things.

Fitting toys that entail trial-and-error practice are needed and greatly enjoyed. It is the baby's striving and succeeding that build his self-image, a feeling of autonomy, and the will to master. It is absolutely necessary that an infant explore tactually what he perceives visually.

Every sensorimotor activity enables an infant to incorporate his learnings into schemata, each one being a sort of personal assimilation of the environment. The baby's ideas are continually modified by fresh data he acquires through each new experience. For example, if faced with a play situation that is novel to him, perhaps getting a watch on a chain out of a covered box with a small elliptical hole on top, the baby may first turn the box over and then try to pull the chain through the opening. He can succeed in pulling up the chain, but the watch may not come out because it remains in a crisscross position. The child possesses only two schemata here: (1) turning the box over and (2) pulling up the chain. He may try to enlarge the elliptical hole but fail. If he tries again, turning the box over and pulling the chain out by accident, the chain may turn and since the watch fits the elliptical opening, out it comes.

Repeated assimilative actions and accommodations to the environment build a child's learning pattern. At five months, if an adult drops an object nearby, the infant will not react. But at six or seven months, when the infant holds an object, lets it fall, and hears it drop, he will search for it with his eyes. After many holding and dropping experiments, he will have a scheme for searching the floor for every object dropped: The existence of an object to a seven-month-old is always directly related to his seeing and holding it.

The following are some toys that your baby will enjoy: Busy Clutch Ball, Nesting Buckets, Bath Harbor, small soft vinyl animals, Plakies, ticking clock, plastic beads and blocks, transparent music box, Busy Box, Busy Gym, sturdy rattle toys, et cetera.

THE SEVENTH MONTH

Motor Development	Language
### Gross Motor	### Vocalizing

Gross Motor

Has good control over body. Can hold head erect at 90-degree position for several minutes at a time; even longer if looking at a parent. Turns over easily.

On back, brings feet to mouth in play.

Pushes up on hands and knees and rocks back and forth. Creeps with object(s) in one or both hands. Goes forward. May crawl. May also locomote by raising and lowering buttocks on back, or by sitting on side of flexed leg, propelling with corresponding hand and opposite leg. Helps in being pulled to stand, keeps legs straight. May pull self to stand.

When supported under arms, stands and bears weight, bounces, steps in place, looks at feet.

Sitting

Sits with light support. Balances well. Hands free while sitting.

Wheels around, leans over. May get self to sit by pushing up with arms from side, or getting into crawl position and sticking out legs in front.

Fine Motor

Thumb apposition complete. Thumb and fingers grasp block.

Uses hands to reach for objects. Grasps object with palm of hand.

Holds two objects, one in each hand, simultaneously; may bang together.

Vocalizing

Vowels and consonants occur at random. Has special, well-defined syllables, usually four or more; most common sounds like "ma," "mu," "da," "di," "ba." Says several sounds in one breath.

Language development begins in earnest.

Tries to imitate sounds or sound sequences.

May say "dada" and/or "mama."

Responding

Listens to own vocalizations and those of others.

Mental	Social
### Sensory Response	### Personal
Sees as well as a teenager. Can locate sounds with amazing accuracy.	Reaches and pats mirror image.
### Attention Span	Explores body with mouth and hands.
Attention more concentrated; interested in detail.	May chew fingers and suck thumb.
### Eye-Hand Coordination	May fear strangers.
Reaches for and grasps toy, like bell or rattle, with one hand. Continues to overextend fingers and concentrate full attention.	Recognizes family members.
	### Interaction
Distinguishes near and far objects and space.	Begins to show humor. Teases. Shows desire to be included in social interaction.
Grasps, manipulates, mouths, shakes, bangs object. Plays vigorously with noisemaking toys like bell, music box, or rattle.	Resists pressure to do something he doesn't want to. Distinguishes friendly and angry talking. May fear performing some familiar activities.
### Memory	May cry when parent leaves. Is choosy about who picks him up. Gives familiar adults hugs and kisses.
Looks briefly for toy that disappears.	
Responds with expectation to the repetition of an event or signal. Remembers segment representative of an entire situation. Remembers small series of actions in immediate past if series includes his own actions.	### Cultural Self-Help/Routines
	Begins finger-feeding. Holds and manipulates a spoon or cup in play. Requires independence in feeding.
	Stays dry one or two hours.
May begin imitating an act.	### Play and Playthings
Continues to compare activities done by one, then the other, side of his body. Visually associates similar acts of his and another person. Responds playfully to mirror image. May associate picture of baby with himself, give appropriate sound.	Wriggles in anticipation of play. Plays with toys.

(continued)

Motor Development	Language

Please do not regard this chart as a rigid timetable. Babies are unpredictable. Some perform an activity earlier or later than the chart indicates.

Mental	Social
Interested in consequences of his behavior. Recognizes an event as a goal only after performing the means.	

Discriminating and Associating

Begins to learn implications of familiar acts. Aware of and compares size differences of similar objects, like blocks.

Transfers object from hand to hand. Retains two or three blocks or small toys offered.

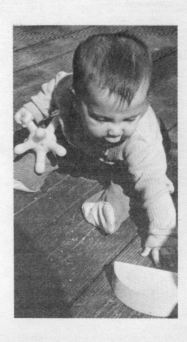

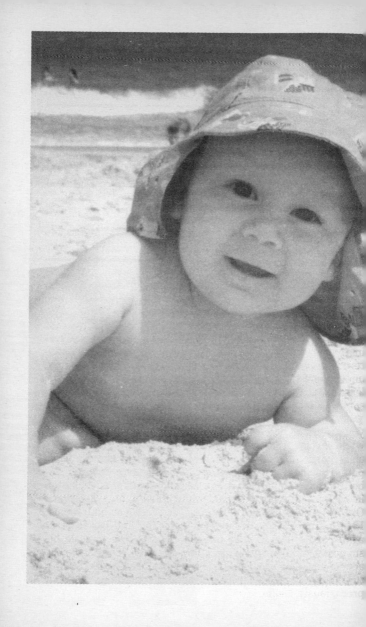

The Eighth Month

MOVING OUT

By this time, your baby will be in perpetual motion when he is awake. He presses forward to new maneuvers, which he joyously combines with his achieved skills. By now he can move well enough to follow you wherever you go. Although he still crawls when he wants to get anywhere quickly, he spends his playtime learning to stand. The baby's steadily increasing ability to get around means that you must strike a balance between containing him and giving him freedom to explore. You must also handle his disinterest in sleep, which limits new and exciting discoveries; understand his fear of strangers; and cope with all the new learning that comes from his added exposure to new sights, sounds, and feelings.

Most babies are developing their upright capabilities. If you watch the process carefully, you will see that your baby, while seated, will spread his feet, draw his knees up slightly, and tug on the side of his crib or any other convenient support until he gets into a flexed, half-standing position, his bottom out and wavering. As he gains control of each step in his pull-up, he is free to recognize and use variations. One is a choice between letting go with one or both hands. If he really lets go, he plumps to sitting and has to start again. If he lets go with one hand, he is free to scale his support hand-over-hand. In a day or so, he coordinates the acts of scaling and rising to full height. Then he learns how to gain his balance after leaning against something, to stand, precariously, alone.

He applies little of this experimentation to sitting. He pivots on his bottom until he is dizzy and falls over, but rarely practices at reversing direction. Since he has mastered the basic skill, sitting is fast becoming less exciting than standing.

Being able to stand doesn't mean your baby is going to know how to get down. Most babies spend several painful weeks learning how. Some try falling backward, but since bending as he falls is very difficult for a baby this age to learn, this "solution" is just too painful. Falling backward also triggers the old, disturbing Moro reflex (the startle reflex), which strengthens the baby's inclination to fall straight back with back arched, arms extended, and head and neck thrown back. Although this often means a banged head, infants don't usually hurt themselves in such falls. Fortunately, their skulls are still flexible and cushion the brain so that falls are less likely to produce concussions than they are in adults. Even so, it would be a good idea to put a rug under large pieces of furniture from which your baby could fall.

If your baby continues to have difficulty in getting himself down from his new standing position, try to teach him. Stand him at your knees, bend him slightly at the middle, and then gently push him forward and down so that he half falls into a sitting position. Doing this several times will eventually give him the idea, even though the first daily session, in which he giggles and thoroughly enjoys your instruction, may make you feel he hasn't learned a thing. After a few days, you may be lucky enough to hear or see him practice his new task. When you know he can get himself down, don't cater to his crying for the same assistance at night. The first few times, reteach him just as you did during the day, then let him get to sleep on his own. In a few nights, he will probably stop crying for you.

Although this may seem unnecessarily "disciplinarian," you should not allow his crying at night to continue. Your tension and fatigue will not be much help to you and the rest of the family, and it could spoil your relationship with your baby. He needs the chance to learn about independence from you in small doses.

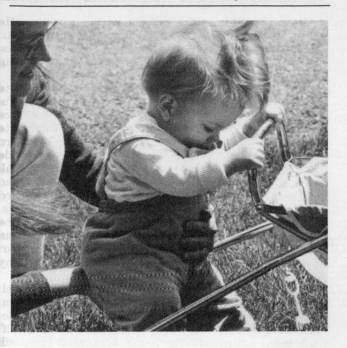

Life is not all mad activity. More quiet experimentation can busy your eight-month-old for hours. You may have noticed, for example, how much your baby enjoys looking at things upside down. In fact, one way to occupy him on the changing table or in his crib is setting pictures upside down at either end of them. This interest continues into walking, when he will walk with his head thrown back. He may be remembering his usual way of looking at the world many months before, when he had to spend so much time on his back. You may also notice your baby sitting and cocking or shaking his head from side to side as he focuses on something in the distance. He is playing with his new awareness that most things keep their size and shape even though his maneuvers, quick or slow, make an object change perspec-

Using Walkers

You may be considering a walker for your baby at this time. A walker does not help a baby develop the strengths and skills that are required in walking. Actually, walkers are of little value. Instead, creeping and crawling need to be fully mastered because they appear to be prerequisites for ongoing motor development. However, there are some babies who skip creeping and crawling and go right into walking once they are able to stand firmly on their own two feet.

tive. As he recovers his balance, the baby may actually laugh at his ability to change his world.

He will also experiment with his hands. Watch your baby examine any household object you've always taken for granted. He looks at it a long time, feels the surface and edges, turns it upside down and sideways, prods it, and drops it just to find out what this three-dimensional object is all about. Putting small blocks or large, colored wooden beads into a large jar, or taking out spools of thread from your sewing box will also fascinate him for hours. He can use either hand. This "pincer" grasp is so new that he practices his holding ability by turning his hands every which way just as he does with other objects of interest. He intently watches his hand as he repeatedly brings thumb and forefinger together. He drops the block on purpose, watches the process, picks it up, drops it—feeling and looking at the new coordination of his muscles. The baby's wonder and delight with his new skill are really appropriate. This separation of thumb and forefinger from the rest of man's "paw" is a great achievement. It allows man a range of manual dexterity from the most delicate sorting of objects to more powerful squeezing or handling of tools. Most eight-month-olds will put down one object before coping with another. But a more precocious eight-month old may be able to handle two objects simultaneously, pick up one block with one hand, another block with the other, and bang them together

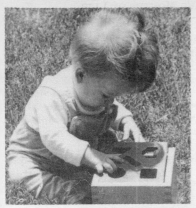

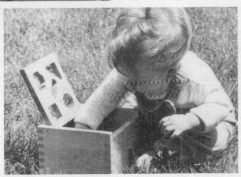

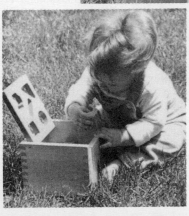

zestfully. If he is really advanced, he may even try reaching for a third block with his mouth, or put one of those in his hand into his mouth and pick up the third with his empty hand.

His intrigue with his own prowess means that he may crawl with one hand filled while he explores with the other. It also means he may begin to empty drawers and cupboards and try tearing things up, including the magazine you haven't read. If your baby manages to acquire a valuable book, don't snatch it away. He may grip it so tightly that you will tear it. Even if this doesn't happen, you will frustrate and bewilder him. Instead, give your baby some magazines of his own to play with. Screen bookcases containing valuable books or art objects with wire mesh when you're not around to protect them. That way he can continue his manual practice, and you can keep your cool, as well as your valuables.

The baby can probably open drawers, too, and one favorite sport may be garnishing the floor with their contents and replacing the original holdings with himself. If you have loop handles on bureaus, dressers, or cupboards, insert a broomstick through them to avoid the inconvenience and mess.

An agile baby is equally able to empty and climb into an older child's toy chest. If it becomes a favorite foray of his, you may have trouble on your hands. The lid can slam over him and trap him inside. Your other child may also rightly resent the invasion of his property. He may fight back, fume helplessly, or if he's especially loving, try teaching his troublesome sib that replacing things can be as much of a game as removing them. As long as he participates, it probably will be enjoyable for the baby. You might help your older child and possibly prevent a tragedy by putting a simple lock on the chest that he can open.

The importance of constant reevaluation of the dangers a baby can maneuver into during these months of exploration cannot be overstressed. Store and lock away medicines in an unreachable place, and take care of heat sources. No book can enumerate for you the many everyday things and places your particular baby will find enticing targets for exploration. You, as the best judge now of your baby's style and interests, will just have to come up with solutions appropriate to your own home. Weighing real danger against the value of your baby's exploration makes some of these judgments very hard. Freedom to explore speeds learning and achievement. If you keep after your baby constantly to stop his "mistakes" and potential "hurts," you will divert his exercise into a testing of you in each situation. He will be more interested in drawing you into his play than in exploring and learning from his own efforts. Here again your feelings make the difference. Some American parents do let their babies try things before imposing a "no" because the attempt will help their baby understand, as well as encourage his exploration. Maybe we do demand too much of a baby when we expect him to comprehend "deep" or "hard" or "burning" without having experienced them himself. Dr. Brazelton writes: "In the highlands of southern Mexico, an Indian mother never stops her baby as he crawls to the central fire. She says, 'He will learn.' He does and must."

Containing an active child at this stage of life is a difficult task. In desperation or because important household chores are being neglected, most parents resort to a playpen. Most such units are devoid of play challenges. The floor area is too small for walking or testing bodily skills. It might be wise to explore the new collapsible fence-type corrals that enlarge play space to four times the traditional playpen.

If there are times when you have to leave the room, take your baby with you or put him in his playpen. Many babies object strongly to being left in their playpens. However, if you keep your baby in the playpen for short periods of time with interesting toys to occupy him, and give him plenty of other time during the day to crawl freely, you need not feel guilty about leaving him there.

Exercising Your Baby

To increase your baby's leg and back flexibility, lay your baby on his back. Holding his legs, lift his buttocks off the floor and gently stretch his legs over his head. Go only as far as your baby's flexibility allows. Hold for a few seconds,

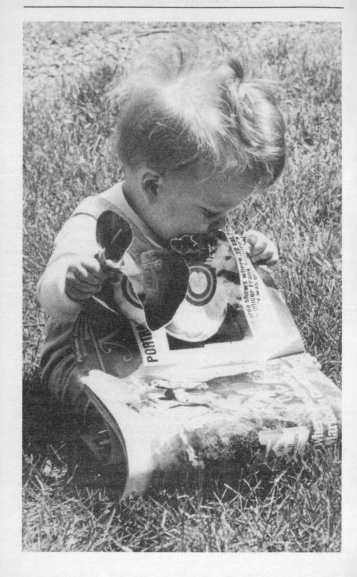

then return his legs to prone position. Repeat gently five times.

To strengthen his arms and legs and hand grip, while in a sitting position on the floor have your baby grab your hands. Slowly raise his arms above his head and lift him to a standing position. After a few seconds, lower his arms and allow his body to return to a sitting position. Repeat gently three or four times.

The Night Watch

Settling down to sleep or quiet times may be equally difficult. Naps may be short and you might have to let the baby give up his morning nap for the single afternoon one. Quiet, sensitive babies, although inactive physically, expend their energy in sorting the kaleidoscope of stimulation they find around them. The sensory and intellectual activity tires them, as does the family hustle and bustle, which is more wearing for them than for more active babies. But an active baby can become so wound up by bedtime that he carries an older child to the point of frenzy with him.

Bedtime is really your decision. It should be handled firmly and with the understanding that few children want to go to sleep. Forcing them to bed may be a relief even to the children because it allows them to quit without losing face. Nothing is as sad as seeing parents wait for their exhausted child to ask for bed. Nine times out of ten, he won't. Children are extraordinarily sensitive to a parent's ambivalence or decisiveness.

Another instance in which you must be decisive is the calling game many babies use when they are at last in bed and don't want to sleep. Unless a parent is firm, the baby may keep calling as long as anyone comes, or keep throwing his stuffed animal over the side and then wailing for its retrieval. Since words in themselves still mean little at this stage, try telling the baby firmly that enough is enough. Put him on his tummy to show him that you don't consider this a fun game.

If a waking crisis begins to occur, you might try a technique suggested by pediatricians. Before you go to bed

Swimming Instruction for Infants

Parents have been getting mixed signals from professionals as to the best age at which to begin swimming lessons for their children. In spite of the warnings of many health and safety authorities, there is a great deal of pressure from parents for swimming instruction for their babies and toddlers. The American Red Cross, National Safety Council, U.S. Public Health Service, American Medical Association, and others recommend that three should be the minimum age for swimming instruction. Parents contend that since water is a baby's natural element, the time to teach swimming is before fear sets in. Not so, say many pediatricians, who maintain that a degree of fear is a necessary safety device to preclude the possibility of accidents in the water.

They believe, too, that babies and toddlers are especially vulnerable to viral infections that can be spread in water. Pool swimming, for example, can increase the incidence of middle-ear infection in young children, and the chemicals in pools present the hazard of the swelling of tissues in the nose and the eustachian tubes.

However, many swimming teachers believe it is important to teach babies and toddlers to swim in order to help protect them from drowning, and because learning to swim is one more step toward building the self-confidence all children thrive on.

To learn about the techniques of teaching swimming to infants, and to help you make up your own mind as to the right age at which to start your child, look for the following books in your local public library:

1. *Teaching an Infant to Swim,* by Virginia Hunt Newman (New York: Harcourt Brace Jovanovich, 1987). Written for parents, this book by a swimming instructor details the process by which she teaches infants to propel themselves through the water and come to the surface to breathe, commonly referred to as the "doggy paddle." Mrs. Newman cautions that parents should check with their pediatrician before beginning any swimming program.

2. *How to Teach Your Baby to Swim,* by Claire Timmermans (New York: Stein & Day, 1975). This well-written book is fully illustrated. A typical lesson includes blowing bubbles (two minutes), floating (five minutes), going under (two to three minutes), floating again (five minutes), jumps (two to three minutes), and more floating (five minutes).

WHAT IS THE BEST AGE TO START TO LEARN TO SWIM?

"The age depends upon the child," say professional swimming instructors. Some babies might be started even at eight months, while other children can wait until they are three years and older, depending upon when the child is going to be exposed to water. If a child is going to be near a pool, a lake, or the ocean, he should be taught to swim at an early age. In any case, at the first sign of discomfort or unhappiness, a baby should be taken out of the water. Learning to swim should be a relaxed and comfortable experience.

SHOULD YOU DELAY INSTRUCTION?

Many experts believe there are definite hazards involved in teaching infants as young as eight months to swim. Even pre-twos are not muscularly able to lift their heads out of water in order to breathe, and are thereby limited to underwater swimming only.

Of course, parents must always remain near young children when they are in or close to water, whether or not they are able to swim. They should never use plastic inflatables and tubes on their children, because they can puncture, thus giving the parents a false sense of security. Should you decide to enroll your child under three in a parent-and-child program, consider it primarily an opportunity for you to enjoy playing in water together and meeting other like-minded parents.

rouse, change, cuddle, and talk to your baby and give him extra milk when he wants it. During the rest of the night, try to ignore him. He will probably awaken a few more nights. But if you tell him firmly that it's sleepy time for him, after a week or so he may need only a pat and a change around ten o'-clock.

The Universe Is Changing Fast

The eight-month-old's increasing ability to move about offers him new vistas of stimulation. The first signs of imitation indicate that your baby is becoming aware of his humanness and sees the similarities between your body and movements and his. When you put on your coat to go out, he begins to cry. Since this act has been followed by your leaving him in the past, he is cleverly anticipating the same sad event.

Watching you imitate *him* adds new consciousness of his own movements that he loves. A mirror hypnotizes him for the same reason. He laughs at the smiling image, pats, and tries to kiss it. He presses his forehead to the mirror to see perhaps if the image is real. He looks at the image of his hand and compares it with the real thing, staring at its changing shapes. The sight of his own body movements enhances the kind of perception, called "visuomotor," that your baby needs to learn physical skills.

Mirror play also stimulates awareness of other infants, because babies usually watch and imitate each other in preference to strange adults. Perhaps infant observers recognize cues from their own repertoires. This awareness of his identity is probably as thrilling to your baby as a new insight about yourself is to you.

By this time, too, a baby is perfectly able to identify a human face. He is looking for new excitement now. Therefore, he will stare at and attend intently representations of new mental models, especially faces of strangers. Dr. Jerome Kagan of the Harvard Center for Cognitive Studies reports that in a series of experiments with strangers and parents in a room with the baby, a nine-month- to fifteen-month-old begins to show fear when parents leave and the stranger remains. This type of encounter shows the first sign of an infant's ability to hypothesize and *think*.

The baby's ability to form mental models is very important. It has been an accurate indicator of intelligence in later childhood, as measured by the best tests available. This ability starts with mother. Her quick and appropriate response to her baby's signals has been experimentally associated with the baby's rapid building of mental models. Deep, eye-to-eye interaction is a basic of the mother-baby relationship and of building a mental model of the human face. Lack of such interaction may be a primary reason why youngsters in institutions can be retarded mentally and socially, especially in their ability to establish and maintain a

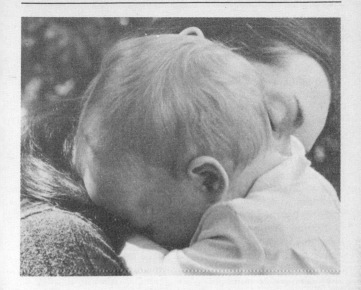

close personal relationship, to profit from past mistakes, and to control behavior for future gains.

The baby's better mobility means he can separate himself from you. He realizes this, and the understanding is frightening. He protects himself from this onslaught by turning to you and away from others, and by being especially fussy when you are near. Even a baby who has been very gregarious will show this new dependence. The baby's increased ability to distinguish himself from others, and family members from strangers, only deepens this awareness. From the time the four-month-old becomes more visually aware until twelve months, his acceptance of strangers drops from about four- to one-out-of-five accepts. Withdrawal from strangers—and that usually means anyone beyond the immediate family—peaks in the next few months.

Suddenly the baby has to be held on your lap during your monthly visits to the pediatrician he's "known" for months. He hates to visit, and doesn't want to be left with the sitter he has had since he was two months old. He weeps as if heartbroken as you leave, although the sitter reports he starts to play when he realizes you are really gone. If you are torn by your "infidelity," do remember that the baby may not be as disturbed as he pretends. Infants can be great actors.

If your baby anticipates your leaving him with a sitter, he may actually stage spitting up his breakfast a few times—just for effect. Instead of scolding him, cuddle him. Tell him you will miss him a lot, that he will have someone to play with and keep him company, and that you will return and have fun together. While what you say will escape him, the warm contact and familiar voice will reassure and comfort him. Gradually, he may be content when you leave and turn to his own activities.

During this period, visits by your friends may provoke frantic embraces, howling, or a more subdued refusal to move or to play with his toys. After the door closes at the end of the visit, *then* your child-wonder will start vocalizing and performing gaily.

Try to prepare your baby before going to a strange place. It's the suddenness of a new experience that frightens him, as much as anything else. Most babies need a bit of time to get acquainted with a strange setup, routine, or person, and you can reassure them. If you notice that your baby is afraid of an object, associate it with something pleasant or look at it, touch it, and handle it together. As you leave home for a visit, talk with him warmly and calmly. Once you arrive, tell your baby repeatedly in a few simple words not to cry, and hold onto him tightly. Suggest to an eager grandparent or aunt not to approach or look at the baby for a little while after arrival, until he approaches them. Looking a baby dead in the eye can build a barrier of wailing as self-protection. Gradual, partial changes are best for a baby, and preparation for the ordeal also helps the relatives. They and other strangers will not feel so bewildered if their eager approaches produce tears and screams, and the baby may soon be able to contain himself to an occasional sob or a stony, anxious silence. Only a well-intentioned chuck under the chin or an overassertive hug will break his resolve and again produce open sobs. However, by the end of the month, he may sit in a relative's lap, poised if not charmingly expansive. When he successfully keeps his cool, you might try a word of praise. He has taken a giant step in social growth.

At home, you may notice that your baby is more anxious at certain times, such as right after a nap when he is not fully awake, or when you are too many rooms away from him. When you are safely nearby, your baby crawls around an obstacle, turns to check on you, looks you in the eye, and then smiles. Out of sight, he maintains a flow of chatter. If you move or stop answering, he will scurry right over and bid for some cuddling. This is suddenly serious play. The meaning of separation is apparent, yet the capacity to separate is fragile. You should encourage these experiments as they will reassure your baby and reinforce his ability to explore without fear.

The baby also needs assurance that you will be there when he returns from his excursions, and that you will be there for *him*. If you pick up a friend's baby and your baby tries to push him out and to climb into your lap, don't tease him. His frantic effort to dislodge a rival is a trauma from which you can spare him. These constant bids may drain you, especially if the baby is your first or your relationship with him is still a bit uneasy. The dependency of a first child is especially wearing because mother or father is new to the job, and because there are no sibs to buffer and diffuse the intense relationship. Parents differ also in their acceptance of this behavior according to where they live. Those in large cities are supposedly less tolerant and push their babies more toward independence. On the other hand, a small apartment only intensifies proximity, and many young parents find their nerves strung out by day's end. Even so, if you really want to foster the very independence that will free you and your baby, let him cling now instead of shoving him away.

The baby's reactions to relatively insignificant separations and upsets are clues to how he would react to major ones. Babies who have to be hospitalized cling and cry desperately. When they return home, they may also eat and sleep badly, vocalize less, and refuse to be distracted from anxiously scanning their homes.

This prewalking period is no time for any unnecessary separation from you or from familiar surroundings, no matter how short. Dr. John Bowlby, a scientist who has done perhaps the finest research to date on the nature of parent and child attachment, says, "The protest, despair and detachment that typically occur when a child over six months is separated from his mother are due to loss of maternal care at this highly dependent, highly vulnerable stage of development. The child's hunger for his mother's presence is as great as his hunger for food, and her absence generates a powerful sense of loss and anger."

He adds that the trauma of early loss or separation from the parent can carry over to produce similar responses in older individuals. Such disturbed adults tend to make excessive demands upon others and, if these are not met, to react with anxiety and anger.

A Certain Style

Although motor skills and fear of strangers are more visible this month, your baby is learning in other important areas also. After all, visual and motor exploration leads to greater familiarization with the environment. It gives the context for all later learned or instinctive behavior. One lesson the baby learns now is the basics of quantity. He places one object after another in a bottle, playing with the concept of "more than one." He shakes the bottle with one object in it to make a rattle. Then he shakes it with several as if to hear the difference. He can pick up objects in each hand, bring one to his mouth, then another, then both as if establishing the difference between "each" and "both" with his mouth. He picks up apple chunks with one hand and banana bits with the other, as if sorting their differences by assigning a hand to each.

He is also developing some complex mental skills, perfecting learning methods, and establishing learning styles that will stay with him for years. He is beginning to make associations with things independent of *his* participation. For example, he crawls to the front door when he hears it open because he has associated its opening with arrivals and

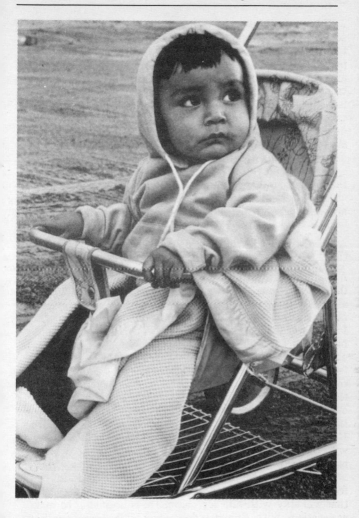

he is a curious creature. He applies the critical mental power of discrimination to an ever-increasing variety of activities and needs.

As early as the first month, your baby could distinguish mother's voice and father's. Now, as he is mastering standing, he is learning to discriminate between pieces of furniture stable enough to support him and those that will topple with him. At first he may pull over anything, his sister's doll table, sofa pillows, or blankets, and fall backward. But after the first trials and errors, he gradually settles down to a few favorite, sturdy spots to which he returns for his daily pull-ups.

His discriminatory power may also serve a real noisemaking urge. First he learns, perhaps accidentally, that if he bangs his hands flat on a tabletop he makes a loud thumping noise. He tries it on any table he finds. Then he figures out that some tables make more noise. He learns that a table full of china rattles especially, so he rushes to the breakfast table after you take him out of his bounce chair. If you doubt that he has associated table and china with more and more intriguing noise, watch his face one morning when you've already removed the cups and saucers.

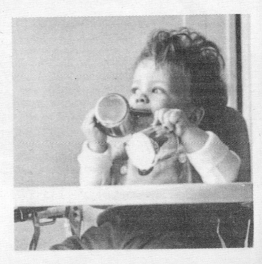

At this stage, your baby develops some complex mental skills, including memory of timing and "gestalt." By gestalt we mean a mental perception of the whole without emphasis on individual parts. For example, if your baby likes to explore rooms, you may notice that a displaced coffee table or a new object gracing the end table attracts him immediately. His memory of the entire scene, or the "gestalt," fixed in this case by his last sight of the room, frees him to efficiently select the new, or discrepant, piece. If your other babies weren't as persistent or alert to detail, this one may surprise you so much at first that the cocktail glasses left from last evening's company may tumble to his charge.

He is also developing a memory of timing. He may terminate a particularly awful feeding by judiciously dropping his cup overboard. As he releases it, he blinks his eyes in delicious anticipation of the cup's crash. He has become conscious of the time interval before contact. In the evening he crawls to the front door to greet his father even before it opens. This may be a first example of your baby's ability to recall a past *event* rather than a past action of his own. His new sense of timing leads him to expect an important, regular event.

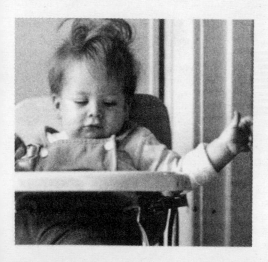

One learning method we all use is to push around our "knowns" until they form a new pattern. The baby does this very early when he climbs. Scaling mammals learn to climb instinctively and unconsciously simply by joining reflexes appropriate and ready for climbing. Although our infants inherit some instinctive urge to climb, the several skills needed for it are *learned* and first used for activities that have nothing to do with climbing. To climb, the baby consciously borrows a known technique here and another there, and eventually puts them together in one smooth performance. First he gives up a two-handed grasp in favor of alternating hands. Then he adds a flexing and straightening of his body to scale upward. He learns to put together segments of a whole action with remarkable speed.

The ways babies put together these basic learning methods to acquire mental skills is as much a part of a personal style as the way each moves. In experiments with one- to ten-month-old babies at Harvard's Center for Cognitive Studies, faces and balls appeared briefly in each of two windows. Some babies found the faces more interesting; some, the balls. Others were equally attracted by both. Reports from parents suggest that, in some cases at least, those who prefer the balls are happier when playing with objects and toys; those who prefer the faces are happier in social interactions.

Some babies will not be pressured to perform before they are ready. This stubborn determination is a kind of strength. Some babies operate with a master plan for reaching their goal. They learn maneuvers separately and put them together deliberately toward an end result. They react more to a situation as a whole. Others have a roster of skills that they sample until they find what works for them. Both types may practice until their self-assigned tasks become "easy"—a quality of persistence essential in moving toward a goal. Still others prefer to manipulate people in their environment instead of working with their own accomplishments. An only child with hovering parents may already know how to play helpless. As a tot, he may continue to point to things instead of naming them because his mother or father has always been his interpreter. The baby may habitually refuse to get his own toys because you have always gotten them. If you notice a clue like this, try some judicious inattention. If you can, get your baby to give up this learning approach. It is probably not rigidly fixed yet.

Constructive molding and teaching imply the parents' appreciation of their baby's learning pace and style. As the late Dr. Lawrence K. Frank of the Macy Foundation put it: "Children have different cognitive styles, their own individual ways of perceiving and understanding the world, some visual, others auditory, while others prefer to deal with the world as it can be directly manipulated and felt. Various studies are showing that once a perceptual style has been developed it resists modification or replacement."

Feeding

The following is a sample one-day menu for an eight- to twelve-month old, as suggested in *Caring for Your Baby and Young Child,* by Steven P. Shelov, with the seal of the American Academy of Pediatrics (New York: Bantam Books, 1991):

Breakfast: ¼–½ cup cereal, ¼–½ cup diced fruit, ½–⅔ cup milk.

Snack: ½ cup apple juice or ¼ cup diced cheese or cooked vegetables.

Lunch: ¼–½ cup yogurt or cottage cheese, ¼–½ cup yellow vegetables, ½–⅔ cup milk.

Snack: ½ cup apple juice or 1 teething biscuit or cracker or ¼ cup diced cheese or meat.

Dinner: ¼ cup diced poultry, meat, or tofu, ¼–½ cup green vegetables, ¼ cup noodles, pasta, rice, or potato, ¼ cup fruit, ½–⅔ cup milk.

Before Bedtime: ½–1 cup milk or water (if milk, follow with water or brush teeth afterward).

Of course, you will check your baby's nutrition needs with your pediatrician or well-baby clinic personnel.

THE EIGHTH MONTH

Motor Development	Language

Motor Development

Gross Motor

Pivots on tummy. Crawls. May go forward or backward at first. May crawl with one hand full. May also go forward by sitting and bouncing on buttocks or by standing, lunging, and grabbing at furniture.

Stands leaning against something, hands free. Pulls on furniture to stand. Needs help to get down from standing. May stand holding onto hand. Held standing, puts one foot in front of the other.

Sitting

Gets self to sit. Pushes up with arms from side; or in crawl position, flexes one leg to tummy, extends and pushes it against surface; other leg follows.

Sits alone steadily with one leg stretched out in front, the other flexed. Sits and bounces on buttocks.

Can sit erect without support for at least ten minutes.

Fine Motor

Thumb, first and second fingers grasp block. Has pincer grasp, thumb and forefinger. Tries to pick up pellet; rakes. Grasps partially with fingers. Picks up string.

Holds rattle for at least three minutes.

Reaches for objects with fingers overextended. Must pay full attention.

Clasps hands.

Language

Vocalizing

Babbles with variety of sounds and inflections spontaneously, for fun or alone; still primarily for self. Imposes adult intonation on babbling. Shouts.

Some eight-month-olds learn "first" words: mommy, daddy, bye-bye, baby, ball, cookie, etc.

Understands simple instructions.

Vocalizes satisfaction.

Begins to mimic mouth and jaw movements.

Uses two-syllable utterances. May label an object in imitation of its sound: e.g, train, choo-choo. May say dada and/or mama as specific names. Increasing repetition of some syllables.

Responding

Usually responds (e.g., turns head and torso) to familiar sounds nearby: his name, the telephone, vacuum cleaner. Listens selectively to familiar words; begins to recognize some.

Shakes head no.

Mental	Social

Mental

Sensory Response

Great interest in cause-and-effect relationships; pulling a string on a crib exerciser and making wheels turn, bells sound, etc.

Attention Span

Reacts promptly to situation.

Eye-Hand Coordination

Examines objects as external, three-dimensional realities. Watches hands in various positions, holding and dropping objects. Explores notions of "in" and "out," "container-contained" by putting small objects in and out of jar. Searches behind a screen for an object if he is looking at it as it is hidden. Only conceives of object in place where it first appeared.

Memory

Recalls past event rather than a past action of his own. Retains small series of events in immediate past without his own action. Anticipates events independent of his own behavior. Begins showing memory of timing; memory of "gestalt." Has mental model of the human face; grows interested in variations of the model. Begins imitating people and behaviors out of sight and earshot.

Social

Personal

Pats, smiles at, tries to kiss mirror image.

Interaction

Fears strangers. Is clearly attached to parents. Fears their separation. Usually awakens or quiets when parent talks to him.

Shouts for attention.

Pushes away something he doesn't want. Rejects confinement. May know how to use parents to get things for him.

Cultural Self-Help/Routines

May have trouble sleeping.

Play and Playthings

Reaches persistently for toys beyond reach. Bites, chews toys. Delights in toys that can be banged, thrown, dropped. Ready for hide-and-seek games. Interested in stuffed animals, balls, nesting cylinders, etc.

(continued)

Motor Development	Language

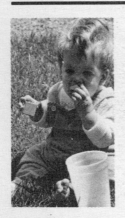

Mental	Social
Body and Object Awareness	

Body and Object Awareness

Aware of the relation between his body and movements and those of others.

Subordinates means to goal. Solves simple problems. Kicks at hanging toy and tries to get it. Rings bell purposefully. Pulls string to secure attached toy.

Discriminating and Associating

Holds and manipulates one object, like a block, and regards second type of object, like a cup. May attempt to secure three blocks. Begins establishing differences between each and both, and between one and more-than-one.

Begins establishing a learning style. Begins using learning techniques. Combines known bits of behavior into a new act.

Please do not regard this chart as a rigid timetable. Babies are unpredictable. Some perform an activity earlier or later than the chart indicates.

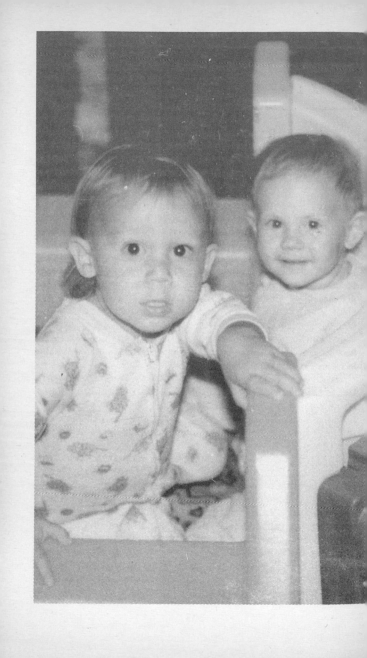

The Ninth Month

UPRIGHT AND FEELING

DOWN

After the tremendous surge of activity in the seventh and eighth months, when your baby perfected his sitting and crawling abilities and began to stand, the ninth month is a temporary slack. The baby uses this period before he walks to secure his impressive gains, to practice mental skills and acquire some social arts. He settles on a definite crawling style, and his speed improves. When the telephone rings he can beat you to it and will listen patiently to the perplexed voice at the other end of the line before you arrive. He is also diverted by just lifting the receiver and listening to the series of developing sounds.

He polishes his sitting performance by rolling smoothly to his side, subtly shifting balance, and continuing on up to sit. Many babies will also sit by getting into a crawl position, flopping back on their bottoms, and bringing their legs out in front. Some babies will get themselves to sit in both ways before settling on one.

The baby's memory and other mental capabilities also improve. In experimental environments, nine-month-olds clearly become bored with, in fact plainly dislike, repetitions of the same stimulation. Younger babies fail to grow bored because each presentation is novel. A nine-month-old can remember a game he's been playing with his sibs the evening before, and will try to get them back to it in the morning. His memory of his pediatrician's office after several months' absence demonstrates recall in an even more important situation. He can now fully conceive of some objects as independent of his ego.

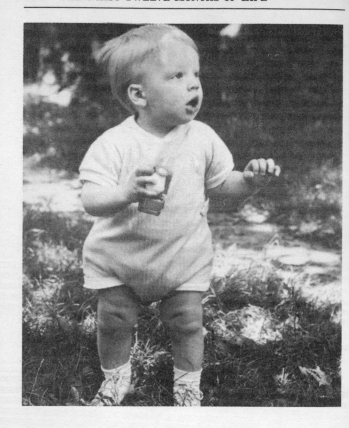

If he can move to a place with one toy, then return repeatedly to get others for his play, he is able to keep a series of ideas in mind. This ability to attend to and use several ideas at once is an important mental skill.

When he can build a small tower of two or three blocks, he is learning more about quantity and the concept of things in a series. He is also acquiring persistence. Without this ability to keep at something until it is done, bursts of artistic inspiration, no matter how brilliant, seldom become achievements for others to enjoy. Equally marvelous is the muscular control necessary to grasp a block with a two-finger grasp, pick it up, convey it to another block, and align the two so they will not topple.

Don't be disturbed if your baby doesn't match these descriptions. Many babies about nine months old, especially very active and very quiet ones, may be devoting themselves to other very different learning tasks. This is perfectly fine and suited to their own growing pace. Differences among babies will be more pronounced now than they were during the first six months of life, when the baby's brain and nervous system were changing more dramatically and his reflexes were more in control of his movements.

A quiet baby may spend part of his day unobtrusively experimenting with all aspects of sitting. He may even propel himself sitting on the side of one leg bent at the knee, pulling with the arm on the same side, and pushing with the foot on the opposite side. This new way to get about may replace his slower belly flops, and his speed increases slowly. In his stroller or walker, he is content to sit and make changes in his visual world by covering his eyes or bending his head at different angles.

By contrast, many a baby may actually stand alone, unsupported. Letting go of his familiar supports, he daringly totters from one leg to the other. A baby often grows quite enamored of a big developmental step such as this. His relentless practice often means that he will greet any limitations of it, including sleep, with resistance. You may have to cut out a nap and try to dress and feed your baby as he stands if he is really insistent. The baby, sitting, crawling, or standing, is now likely to be anywhere in the house, so calling to see where he might be hidden becomes *de rigeur*. In the space of a week or so, an active baby may learn to push himself up from his tummy with both arms, place one foot and then the other on the floor, straighten his legs and arms, and come to stand *by himself* by lifting his trunk and using his waist as a pivot. He may stop the action at one point in the routine and crawl like a spindly daddy longlegs, bottom high in the air, on his straightened arms and legs.

A very active baby may even want to take steps holding onto your hands, or actually lunge from wall to wall or furniture in his desperation to get moving. This month may also

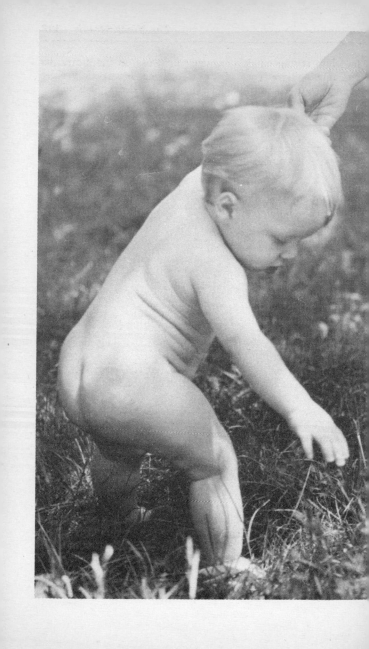

find him trying out his crawling prowess on the stairs, so you must either teach him how to back down safely if he doesn't figure it out himself or make the stairs off-limits.

A New World

With the ability to stand comes a price tag of insecurity and the job of reappraising old skills that suddenly have other dimensions and new implications. The baby becomes aware of vertical spaces as he climbs up and down from heights posed by chairs and stairs.

He also learns a sense of space from using his hands more and more efficiently. He begins to accommodate his hands to the shape of what he is reaching for. He grabs for a large, round object with both hands as if he knows he needs both to hold it. He turns his hand so that he can pick up a pencil along its long dimension.

He is suddenly afraid to budge from chairs he has climbed from many times before, and he may be concerned about as simple a thing as a vacuum cleaner. When you turn it on, he cries miserably in a corner. Since he is probably intrigued as well as terrified, leaving him in another room is no answer. Instead, hold him close with one hand while you vacuum with the other and calmly say something like "It won't hurt you." When the vacuum is turned off, encourage him to touch and explore it. Gradually the baby will conquer this dread, too, and play comfortably as you work. Another new fear may be the bathtub. He may have been playing in it for months, yet now he whimpers pitifully during his bath and clutches the tubside passionately. Bathe him in his old bathinette if it makes him happier, or bathe him with you in the tub, holding him close as you lower him. He will slowly regain his old confidence and in a month or so feel up to taking a bath alone again.

He may also have trouble getting along with his brothers and sisters. Babies, even those used to fielding the noise and commotion of sibs, show increased sensitivity to children during this period. Their vigorous, unpredictable movements and sounds are just too much to tolerate as the baby conquers new fears and insecurities.

Even though sibs may seem an added hardship during this period of readjustment, the baby's constant work and interest in mastering all that happens around him attest to the worth of a stimulating environment. A baby who sees few children besides a brother or sister is especially sensitive to other children now. An only child may be so unused to them that he stares uncooperatively as they play nearby, jumps if they move or shout suddenly, or shrinks away fearfully if they approach him. This kind of baby actually needs more contact with children to overcome his sensitivity. A baby *is* more interested in watching children than adults, and babies in preference to older children. If your baby is socially inexperienced, allow him to take in his universe slowly. Two or three active youngsters in his own house at the same time may present too big a slice of life at this stage of his growth.

How Parents Can Help

Parents react differently to a baby's fear. Some parents overreact and are too protective. Others push too hard and even resent the baby's old attachments. Parents with more than one child are particularly prone to this. Suddenly aware of something about the baby they think needs attention, their guilt about imagined neglect pushes them. For example, all the babies in the neighborhood are using a cup by now, so mother grows exasperated at her baby's clumsiness and determines to wean him from his bottle with which he is content. Some of her neighbors agree with her. The baby, however, resists these efforts. The more she presses, the more determined he becomes. When she "cons" him with flavoring, he drinks milk from his cup, but when she phases out the flavoring, he balks again. The baby may cue her to his feelings in other ways. Milk from the cup rolls down his face while orange juice, for instance, is swallowed neatly.

Try imitation to teach your baby to manipulate and drink from his cup. Give the baby a cup while you use one. Then give him some milk to experiment with. Let him play with his cup in the bathtub, where he cannot create a mess, even if he does sample the bath water, too. If you make using a cup a game, the baby will learn how to use it unaware, and the real transition from bottle to cup will be less painful.

Appropriate comfort and reinforcement are most important during this stage of your child's life, but they are not easy. Each incident demands an on-the-spot evaluation and a prompt response. You can probably hearten a baby more easily with a kind word and a gentle squeeze if you respond to his cry immediately. He is more likely to dissolve into a quivering heap of self-pity if you wait too long.

Another way to help is to turn a fear into a positive experience. A baby may be in such a hurry as he crawls that he gets ahead of himself and falls forward on his nose. His pained look may reflect more surprise at his predicament than real hurt. You can boost his morale with a quick hug or a sympathetic pat on the back, and by calmly setting him straight again. Short and sweet, these boosts might do better than prolonged expressions of sympathy. With prompting from a few minor accidents at which you laugh, the baby may sprawl deliberately on his tummy and face and squirm with laughter—strictly for your benefit. Your amusement encourages his budding sense of humor.

Language Learning

Toward the end of the eighth month and in the ninth, a baby's repetitive babbling is strung together into drawn-out phrases of four or more syllables, for example, "loo-loo-loo-loo-loo." Now the infant ceases to repeat the same sound over and over; instead he combines different sounds so that he may say "ad-dee-dah-boo." Once this combination appears, he is on the verge of producing his first words. His inflections become so marked and varied that he sounds as if he were talking fluently but in another language. Henceforth, his vocalizations are decidedly influenced by his language community.

Showing, Shaping, and Shoving

Because your baby is becoming more and more of an individual in the ways he does things, your help and intervention need to become more specialized. Dr. Gewirtz says that many parents do not understand the importance of the circumstances in which such things as food and love are provided, particularly as these circumstances relate to the baby's behavior. Research at Harvard's Center for Cognitive Studies indicates that clumsy intervention that violates the child's cycle of effort and pause can bring frustration, failure, and tears. Harvard researchers asked mothers to help their six-month-olds fetch a toy from behind a transparent screen. Since babies this age do not solve this task spontaneously, the mother's style of assistance was important. Kenneth Kaye, who conducted the research, picturesquely calls the three teaching techniques he distinguished "showing, shaping, and shoving." In the first, the mother shows the baby what to do. He found that mothers do this when they believe, rightly or wrongly, that the baby can organize a comparable act although the baby may not have shown that he could do more than parts of it. "Shoving" was literally guiding or pushing the baby's hand. It grew from the mother's conviction that the infant already knew how to do the job well. "Shaping," the most sophisticated teaching method, involved breaking down the act into more manage-

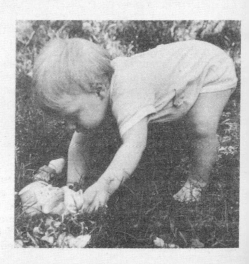

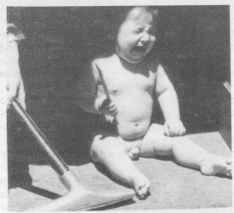

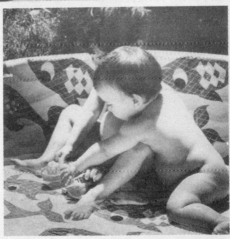

able segments, the basic idea behind programmed learning. For example, the mother first moved the toy to the edge of the screen so the baby could reach and grab, minus the difficult cues of transparent materials and the complicated problem of hooking his hand behind something. Mothers used this modeling technique when they felt the baby was not quite up to the task. Wrongly applied, each teaching technique led the baby to resist, avert his eyes, and break off the learning exchange with his mother. Appropriately applied, each technique was successful. One critical requirement for success was the mother's timing so that her teaching occurred during the natural breaks in the baby's activity. Another was the mother's correct judgment of her baby's cues. For example, a mother could think her baby able to do a task when in fact he was not up to it and, therefore, would shove him rather than shape his behavior.

Generally, a parent's teaching should grace the baby's readiness for a learning task and aim to support his self-realization, neither ignoring nor overwhelming it. The baby will add voluntary mastery to his system of reflexes, at a time when freedom and exploration can characterize his achievements. Then a baby can refuse as well as accept what he is about to internalize. When he can accept it, he experiences the sheer joy of learning that will enrapture you when your baby first walks. These feelings are reason enough. But additional bonuses in this teaching style are the greater stability of the behavior itself, easier teaching, and your satisfaction in teaching successfully.

Self-Help

Besides your intervention, the baby himself will try to cope. He may act out some of his new fears, experiences, and goals. If you look for them, you will see these precious bits of play and practice. For example, he may try to allay his anxiety about heights by repeatedly standing, then purposely falling to his knees or bottom. He may crawl up a few stairs, drop his favorite stuffed animal down them, then crawl back down to the bottom, pick it up, and console it. This is an early sign of symbolic thought. The baby has clearly recorded a situation in his mind so effectively that he can "put it on" to something else. For example, after a trauma like hospitalization or even a visit to the dentist, an older child will often ease his scars with play, repeatedly acting out bits and pieces of the experience. If you feel your child needs it, you can even set up a play situation aimed at a difficult episode or an old fear.

With such "self-help" this period is bound to pass. While the baby's fears lead to a temporarily greater need for his mother, they also foretell bursts of independence and growth. They signal that he is consolidating tenuous "feelers" and gathering security from the physical world—and you—before trying new exploits.

There is little real need for friends' advice to determine your handling of your baby. You know yourself and your baby better than anyone else. Sometimes even well-intentioned people are just plain wrong. As Dr. Gewirtz writes: "A parent labeled loving by his community might dispense stimulation which would appear to him and it to indicate love and attentive care, but which may have little or no effect on his child's behavior. On the other hand, the apparently indifferent parent may respond sparingly to his child but the stimulation provided could suit and encourage the child's learning."

We all seem to make the general mistake of equating successful parenting with the child's speed in growing up. Hopefully today's generation of young parents will understand more fully that a wiser aim is soundness, not speed, for each step of child-rearing, and that "doing your own thing" is better than worrying about other people's opinions.

Sibling Rivalry

The time when your baby learns to stand and walk is a common second peak for sibling rivalry. The baby is better able to get in his sib's way and he is becoming a personal threat as well. Just as you could not trust your toddler's feelings during the previous period, you cannot now, especially since his own interim learning may inspire him to even more sophisticated torture methods.

Rivalry between a baby and a toddler can be suppressed or quite visible. You may become aware that your three-year-old is feeding the baby a varied menu of leftovers, birdseed, and aspirin that he wouldn't dare eat himself. These clandestine feedings represent a mixture of unconscious emotions and deliberate intent. Unknowingly, he may even wish to hurt him.

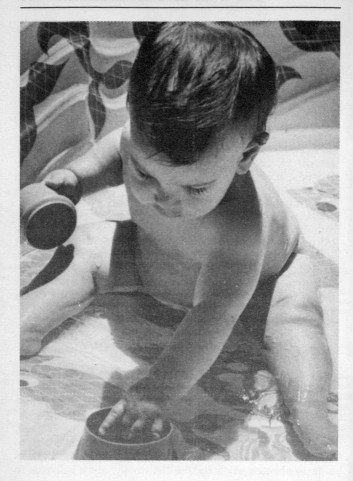

Your toddler may also intervene directly to counter an act that threatens him. As the baby makes a play for your spouse at day's end, your three-year-old butts in and roars to drown out the baby's greetings. Or, realizing how precarious the baby's new standing skill is, your three-year-old skims past him, whirls, and charges during the baby's exercise sessions. The baby falls or grabs that table he's been smart enough to stand close to. Littering the floor around the baby, yelling, or slamming doors—preferably in his face—are other harassments that stem from jealousy.

This unsettling influence retards the standing and walking of many second or third children. Luckily, however, the environment is not wholly responsible for a baby's learning, and baby's inner drive is very strong.

While the baby practices his physical accomplishments, he learns to protect himself and his possessions from a marauder. He begins to gather toys in his lap and hover over them during his brother's bad moods. In the evenings, when his brother sweeps past him to a parent, shoving him in the rush, he flattens to his tummy, hands over his lowered head. He becomes sensitive to his brother's anger and learns to differentiate it from the less dangerous anger of others. He knows when and how long to play quietly in a protected nook or near another family member. And he also grows sensitive to the controls older family members exercise to reduce his danger.

Even though your children's tensions and ugly emotions can be very difficult to handle, fighting has a certain value. Children really enjoy many of their squabbles and fights. When else in their lives will they ever be allowed to release anger so directly? More important, they, like adults, sometimes need to express the ugly side of a relationship to free positive feelings for each other.

The baby learns more from his sibs than the arts of protecting himself and evaluating people's moods and motives. He learns how to cooperate and to live with others. Games, like sports later on, are good outlets for the aggressive, competitive facets of their relationship, as well as a way to learn teamwork. Your baby's wish to appeal to his sib sparks a game of catch. Although he can't really get a ball back to his teammate, he does grasp it with one, then two hands and pushes it out and drops it as if he understands the process. His aim is hardly an asset either, but his brother's pleasure in throwing to the baby motivates him to run and pick up the ball for him. Another ball game can involve throwing a toy for the baby to fetch, even if it also includes grabbing the toy from the baby's hand. A parent should encourage rather than interrupt these healthy exchanges among the children. Dashing to safeguard your baby's right to the retrieved object will only make your two-year-old feel guilty for having snatched it, spoil a valuable exercise, and cast it in another light for both. As is, the game satisfies your baby's love of action and reconciles your toddler's conflicting feelings toward his younger sib.

Babies learn still more from brothers and sisters. Their make-believe tea parties foster the baby's dexterity as he holds his hands and cup in readiness for the promised tea. He learns the social nature of mealtimes. If you give your children a little milk in their cups, your baby may actually learn to drink from a cup during this play.

An older sister and her baby brother may look at picture books and magazines together, if she enjoys them. She may try reading to the baby, who unappreciatively snares the pages and rips them as he tries to turn them too. As your tot murmurs lengthy sentences in imitation of you, she moos for the cows, meows for the kittens, and labels them all. Besides the togetherness, this is valuable language practice for toddler and baby alike.

The relationship among sibs, despite troubled times, is too valuable to sacrifice to your fears of letting them work out their struggles. Unfortunately, many parents feel that after a toddler has won the first round against negative feelings, a rematch is out of order. This reaction only drives hostility underground and makes the older child miserable and possibly even more determined to undermine the baby. These parental expectations are unfair, too, because competitive, selfish feelings are never completely controlled in adults, let alone in children.

BECOMING A SOCIAL BEING

Even at nine months of age, the baby himself is not as helpless as he may seem. As long ago as the 1930s, John Watson, one of the first developmental psychologists interested in babies, researched the way infants played with their contemporaries at different age levels during the first year. Before four or five months, he says, babies hardly seek social contact with other babies although social relationships with adults are already forming. At about five months, one baby will smile to another or cry if another receives attention. But these are courtesy gestures, still removed from real social exchange. Watson put babies six months and over in playpens with toys—hollow cubes, drums and drumsticks, and balls, which the babies were shown how to roll back and forth to each other.

Babies six to eight months old often paid more attention to their surroundings than to the toys or their playmates. When one baby tried to be sociable, the other often ignored him. Friendly contacts, when they did occur, were awkward, almost bashful, and limited to looks, smiles, and mutual grasping. Games were few and short, often consisting of the babies' unspecific handling of the same object. Fights were equally impersonal, more like blind attempts to get

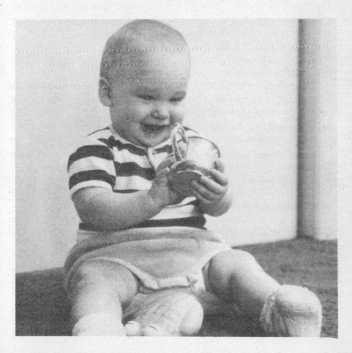

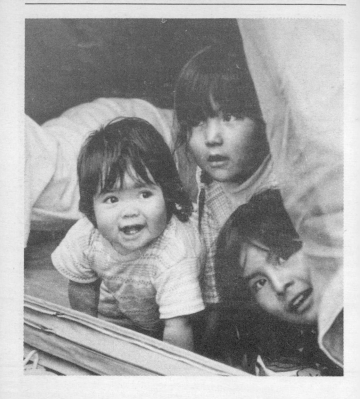

hold of the toys. In contrast, babies nine to thirteen months old responded quickly to the toys. But they were hardly sociable creatures. Since their playmates often became an obstacle to getting them, personalized fighting was at its maximum during these months.

Along with this intensified fighting, your children will come to find more genuine pleasure in each other. Although your older child may be openly antagonistic and competitive as the baby guards himself and his toys, he also begins to respect him as a person for they have begun to play as equals.

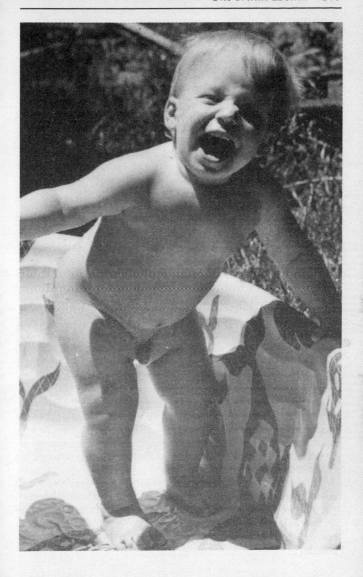

THE NINTH MONTH

Motor Development	Language
### Gross Motor	### Vocalizing
Crawls with one hand full. Can turn around. May crawl upstairs. May crawl on straightened limbs.	Intonation patterns become distinct.
Walks while adult holds hands.	Signals emphasis and emotions by vocalizing.
Stands briefly with hand held. May stand alone briefly. May get self to stand without pulling up on furniture. May sidestep or "cruise" along furniture.	Imitates coughs, tongue clicks, hisses. Uses words meaningfully; says "dada" and/or "mama" as specific names. May say a syllable or a longer sequence repeatedly.
Pulls self to standing.	
### Sitting	### Responding
Sits well in chair. Sits down after standing.	Listens to conversations, singing tones. May understand and respond to one or two words other than name, like no-no. May carry out simple commands; pleased with his understanding, e.g., "Go get my slippers, please."
Sits steadily and indefinitely alone. Pivots 90 degrees seated.	
Gets self to sit effortlessly.	
Can straighten back from forward position.	Responds to his name.
### Fine Motor	
Successfully grasps pellet or shoelaces with thumb and forefinger. Palmar and plantar grasp reflexes disappear.	
Clasps hands or bangs objects together at center of body.	
Index finger begins to lead; points; tries to poke into holes, hooks and pulls.	

Please do not regard this chart as a rigid timetable. Babies are unpredictable. Some perform an activity earlier or later than the chart indicates.

Mental	Social
### Sensory Response	### Personal

Mental

Sensory Response

Fears heights. Aware of vertical space. Recognizes dimensions of objects.

Attention Span

May refuse to allow self to be distracted. May begin showing quality of persistence.

Capable of retrieval memory.

Eye-Hand Coordination

Approaches small object with two fingers, large object with both hands. Changes dimensions of objects by partially covering eyes or looking upside down.

Fingers holes in pegboard.

Uncovers toy he has seen hidden.

Memory

Grows bored with repetitions of same stimulation. May remember a game from previous day. Anticipates reward for successful completion of act or command. Anticipates return of person or thing he has released manually or visually.

Can keep a series of ideas in mind.

Body and Object Awareness

Picks up and manipulates two objects, one with each hand. Hits or pushes objects against each other.

Discriminating and Associating

Drops one of two blocks to get a third. May put one of two objects in mouth and get a third.

Social

Personal

Recognizes mother and self in mirror.

Perceives mother as separate person; father, probably.

Interaction

Anticipates mother coming for feeding.

Entire social life revolves around the primary caretaker.

Performs for home audience. Repeats act if applauded.

May learn to protect self and possessions, fight for disputed toy. May be more sensitive to other children; cries if they cry. Begins to evaluate people's moods and motives.

Shows interest in other people's play.

Cultural Self-Help/Routines

Feeds self cracker. Holds bottle. Uses cup handle. Manipulates and drinks from cup.

May fear bath.

Play and Playthings

Initiates play. May play out new fears. Plays pat-a-cake, so-big, bye-bye, ball games. Chooses toys deliberately. May build tower of two blocks.

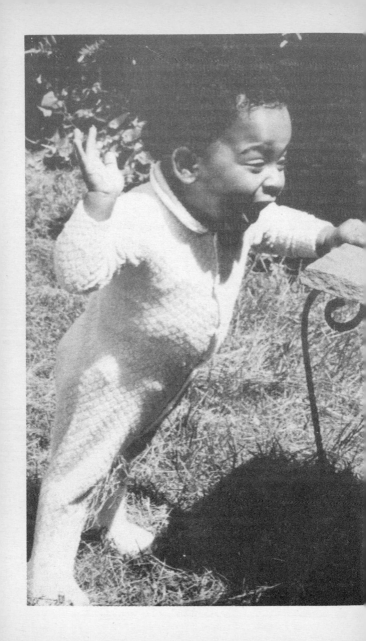

The Tenth Month

IMITATION

In the next several months, your baby will work on putting his world in motion. Unless he is very active, his slowdown in motor learning will very likely continue this month but the lull is deceptive, for he is really gathering strength to carry him through that big step of walking. This month, however, he will expend some of his energy on improving old skills, but he will devote more and more of it to social and personal growth.

He can finger-feed so well now that he can feed himself an entire meal. He is very insistent on feeding himself, although he may still allow you to feed him mushy foods with a spoon. If he has sibs, he will try to keep up and eat with them—the same food, please, in bite size.

He smoothes rough edges off the motions of sitting, crawling, and standing he has so recently and relentlessly learned. He may even get himself to stand by straightening his four limbs from a crawl position, pushing off with his palms, and lifting the weight of his trunk. Standing, he may practice stepping sideways facing a couch. At first hesitant, he "cruises" more and more easily and quickly. Speeding along, he slides one foot after the other, his hands barely skimming the surface of the couch seat. When he learns to walk, he will lose this ability. Keep in mind that many babies, particularly heavy ones, will cruise later, and some never experiment with cruising or standing. They just seem to wait until they can get up and walk.

Cautious about heights in the month before, a ten-month-old dares to climb from a chair now, but still scrupulously

323

surveys the distance. Babies at this age still distrust their visual cues. Brazelton says, "Those who want to slide off an unfamiliar changing table will drop their legs over first to test the space and cling to their support until they feel the ground below." If they can't find it, they scramble up onto the table again. This caution is absent in babies who are hurtlers, but more cautious infants show a respect for heights.

New skills your baby probably will work on are manual, perhaps carrying two small objects in one hand across a room to their container. You may also notice that your baby is beginning to separate the assignments of each hand—the left for carrying and the right for manipulating, if he is "right-handed." Seated, he sucks his left thumb but frees his right for play and exploration. The reduction of the left hand to container and carrier enforces the increasing emphasis and dexterity of the right hand, and begins differentiating active and passive sides of the body. The baby might also be ready to learn the subtleties of pushing an object to one side instead of shoving it forward and backward, his natural style of pushing. Try working with him on a merry-go-round toy. Besides pushing differently, he will also have to discover how and when to let go.

A Late Weaning Means Catching Up

Unlike most babies, a quiet baby may show a long-awaited spurt in motor activity this month. For a quiet baby who may still be nursing, this late spurt in development may prompt a weaning. Physical progress and refusing the breast are often more than coincident. At this time, the baby may wean himself very simply and much more easily than you can. One day, perhaps after a particularly large dose of milk from his cup, he will just avert his face and push your breast with the flat of his hand. There is no denying the meaning of this cue. You shouldn't feel rejected or angry or guilty when your baby first refuses your breast. Your baby may almost imperceptibly show you in other ways that he misses the closeness of nursing times.

You need not worry that you have been constraining your baby's development by nursing him so long. Even though many babies seem swathed in a gentle cocoon during nursing, this period allows the baby to store energy and experience that far outweigh any delay. Maturation of the nervous system doesn't stop in the cocoon. It continues on to certain necessary minimum levels of maturity that allow major developmental events to occur. A three-month-old baby, for example, simply has not reached the minimum level of maturity and muscular control for holding a marble between his thumb and forefinger. When an infant reaches the appropriate stage for a given development, such as sitting up alone, it gets done with very little practice. Children hospitalized with body casts who have never walked can walk within a few days after the casts are off if they have reached the appropriate stage of maturation.

Very quickly, your baby will sit alone, stand, and crawl. He can now sit with a straight back and pivot 90 degrees if he wants to reach for or look at something behind him. His thumb-sucking and sitting will quickly yield to crawling and standing, as if he feels a new freedom at last. Since some quiet babies require a little more encouragement, you may teach yours to stand by firmly refusing to give him a favorite toy you are holding even though he points and calls for it. The incentive of frustration may finally make him creep to you, pull on your legs, grab for your outstretched hands, and pull up, though he may still whimper to be let down. Heartened by his standing successes, he may also begin to crawl. Once he gets going, you may see him head toward a corner to curl into or a chair to huddle under. There he turns to survey the room he has just conquered. Since he doesn't know how to crawl backward yet, you may sometimes have to extract him from between pieces of furniture or from between wall and love seat, where he is firmly wedged, wailing. Despite this inconvenience and his laborious style, the sight of your baby moving may seem more gratifying than anything you've felt in a long time. Even though he is crawling and standing with support at ten months, in comparison to the "average" baby at eight months and a precocious one at seven, remember that he has put three major acts together—sitting, crawling, and standing—in about half the time. He is on his own personal timetable of sturdy development.

In sharp contrast, an active baby may pass most of his time on his feet and protest lying down. A very active baby may even be learning to walk. You will find on your next trip to your pediatrician that all this standing has made the baby lose about an inch of his height. Actually the vertebrae in his backbone have settled. Even adults measure an inch shorter normally than they would if they were bedridden— a small price for being upright.

Tension is often the companion of bursts of physical activity, and this can mean sleeping problems. But unlike earlier periods of unrest, your baby, now physically stronger, can rock his crib on hands and knees and make a racket loud enough to rouse the entire household. You will help everyone concerned by helping the baby with his sleeping problem. Try a little after-dark communion in which you rock and croon to him, and feed him close to you until you feel him begin to let go. It will help him stay asleep later.

A Sense of Identity

During these next couple of months, many babies concentrate on the interaction between their emerging personalities and their families. Your baby will show many real moods and emotions now, and grow more and more self-conscious and aware of social approval and disapproval.

As you know, your baby's crying was his earliest and most easily identifiable emotional response. One reason the baby learned to cry was to signal for your help with his pain or discomfort. But he often cried just to relieve internal pressure, as all advocates of "a good cry" already know. Although he still cries for these reasons, he does so less often. Most likely your baby cries now because of his fear of strange people, places, and activities, or his unhappiness at being separated from you and other loved ones. Even emotional separations, such as the aftermath of a scolding, can make him look sad and hurt. He can sit daydreaming as if he has much to contemplate. He can also grow angry, especially when you frustrate an activity he feels is important. Just like adults, babies get angry more often when they are tired, hungry, or physically not up to snuff. Just like adults, they are more content when they are rested, healthy, and well fed. Your baby's laughter and joy are a delight to the whole family. He shows his pleasure when father or mother comes home in the evening, and he licks his lips in satisfaction at a good meal. He may begin to enjoy music. A familiar tune can set him rocking as he pats his hands and hums along.

Your baby probably extends his tenderness now to stuffed animals and other toys. The capacity to love or mother something is a real compliment to you, for it can come only from the experience of being lovingly and happily nurtured.

The baby also grows sensitive to social approval, partly because of his new awareness that mother and father are humans separate from himself. He can begin to infer something about his parents' goals for him and about the plans

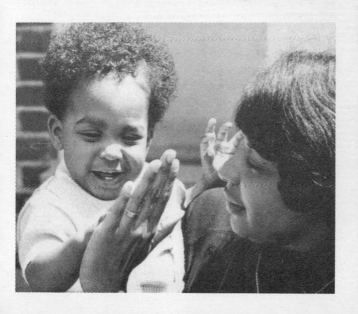

they are adopting to achieve them. Then he can try to accommodate them and win approval, or alter their goals toward his wishes through gentle persuasion or obstinate refusal.

Most babies this age will not show off their latest accomplishments away from home. Depending on his personality, your baby may relish or feel quite shy about performing for a family audience. Capitalizing on his performing arts, his sibs may make him a willing mouthpiece. After he has learned a new word or gesture, your baby may spend days rehearsing it and offering it to every one of your questions. Soon the word loses meaning and appropriateness. It becomes a companion of play, a sound to fill in silence, or a ploy to attract your attention. It lasts as a focal point in time and space as long as you react. When he senses you are growing bored, your baby will discard the mangled word and move on to a new one. In this way, he learns to "look sad," to "snuggle and kiss," and to say "bye-bye," waving as you leave the room or house and giggling and clapping when you return.

On the other hand, your baby may be suspicious of your teasing him. Although he may eventually gain enough confidence to perform at your knee, his attempts are still very fragile. If you laugh, catch his eye, join in the funny little croaks that sometimes sound like a singer's crooning, or try to show him off for anyone else, he stops the recital.

He is also beginning to say no. Sometimes he accompanies his refusals with a wag of his head. Don't immediately assume the baby is being difficult. Even though he can balk when he wants to, the baby probably has only a vague sense of what the word no is all about. Besides, the most natural movement of the head is from side to side, something the baby has been doing since he was a week old, when he followed moving objects with his eyes. So he will learn this gesture more quickly than the nod that goes with yes.

During this emotional growth, the baby is developing his sense of identity about himself and what belongs to him. He may grow disinterested in his sister's toys and play more with his own. He may even be able to sort his own toys from a jumble in the nursery.

His first reactions to himself were probably long-ago percepts of his own body. He heard his own cry, felt his body moving, saw and manipulated his own fingers and toes. Later he learns to recognize his own voice or touch or face as different from those of others. Maybe as late as two years of age, children have some grasp of the total self-unity. At this age, when you ask him, "Where are your ————?" he can point to his teeth, eyes, ears, hair, and toes. You might begin the game by pointing to and naming each part of a favorite doll. Then, as you label, your baby learns to point. After several rounds, you ask the baby where his eyes are. He may be able to point correctly. The ability to extrapolate from the doll to himself is a big step. It means the baby has recognized the doll as an inanimate object that is separate from him, yet with certain clear similarities to his own body parts. If you ask him to point to *your* eyes or nose or mouth, he may show he understands your request by looking at the right feature but turning away, chagrined. Don't be too disappointed at the refusal; his behavior might mean that he recognizes how different you are from him and his doll. Some babies, on the other hand, do better starting with mother's, father's, or a family member's features.

Babies may also start to evolve a sexual identity. Baby boys and girls have differed importantly much earlier than this. Girls are much more consistent in their behavior than boys are, and are generally much more attentive. They are usually more precocious in their development, and are more intrigued with novelty. They also talk more. In experimental situations, baby girls as young as six months of age paid more attention to male than female faces, while their male contemporaries attended more to pictures of females. Now the differences are even more apparent.

Sexual identity probably begins as simple imitation, but is so strongly encouraged by both parents alike that they contribute to its growth. Dr. Howard A. Moss of the National Institute of Health has established experimentally what many social scientists have known for a long time: Parents respond very differently to baby boys and girls. Both mothers and fathers use many more terms of endearment when addressing their baby girls. When parents were requested by researchers to "get their infant to smile and to vocalize," fathers and mothers expended much more effort trying with their baby girls. Since baby boys and baby girls do not differ in their basic ability to smile or vocalize, inborn skills are not what prompt differences in parents' participation.

The Power of Imitation

Imitation begins to play an important role in your baby's learning now. It is a wonderful way to learn. Even a baby who has never before learned a piece of behavior by watching someone else will do so at this stage. Although still very fragile, you can use imitation in your baby's *second year* to institute toilet learning, toothbrushing, and washing the hands and face. Don't be tempted to push it too hard now because you recognize its potential for learning. Parents who *have* pushed have found that their babies' imitation vanished.

Your baby usually will have no qualms about spontaneously identifying with your behavior. He will try to feed you pieces of food, as you have fed him. If you accept them, he is thrilled, laughs when you smack your lips, and watches your chewing and swallowing intently. He dabs at his face with a washcloth in imitation of your washing, and laughs when you imitate his posture and movements after him. When you take your baby from the bathtub and say "brr" and shiver as you dry him, the baby will laugh and try imitating you. As he imitates, he learns some things about cold—the feeling of being chilled, and the way people react to it physically and vocally.

Believe it or not, he will begin picking up some of your less stellar traits as well. If you are compulsively clean, he may swipe away at his feeding table with a towel in imitation of your cleaning gestures. He will spill very little as he brings his spoon to his mouth, and zealously dab his mouth or the tray when he does. Sometimes this isn't good. Babies are naturally messy and precise neatness is unusual at this age. Some baby girls, more than baby boys, show this, but they really aren't old enough to understand the meaning of cleanliness as we do. If a child senses you are upset at his messiness, he may conclude that he must become antiseptically clean; he may get pretty compulsive himself and very upset when he gets dirty. Then he may be afraid to explore the world freely the way a baby usually does to get acquainted with it.

A baby also imitates other babies. On some days in a doctor's office, a baby can initiate a chorus of crying or laughter by this imitative contagion. If you visit another family with a baby, yours may appear engrossed, though removed from the other baby's activity. When you return home, you may see yours imitate the other's play as if he has learned it all. A precocious ten-month-old is perfectly capable of removing the rings from the tower color cone he never played with before and piling them back on their spindle exactly as he saw the other baby do. Twins are especially fine mimics. Often one twin is the doer and the other watches. The "watcher" can suddenly perform in full a routine that his twin has spent days mastering.

Representational memory—memory of behavior and of things seen but out of sight—is the basis of imitation and something else related to it, which psychologists call "object permanence." The baby can retain events for longer and

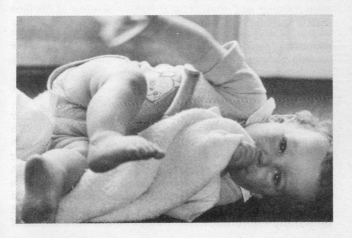

longer periods. He is just beginning to recognize that time is a medium in which he, as well as objects, can be located in relationship to each other.

Memory for what is out of sight grows together with understanding of distance and depth to help the baby imitate behavior and understand the nature of objects. Now he can reach behind himself for a toy as he sits, without turning to look at it, because he has learned that an unseen object has not necessarily disappeared, and he has discovered how to gauge the distance between himself and an object he wants, even with his eyes averted or closed. Not-so-near space isn't a single flat plane anymore, either. The baby's eye and mind can perceive it ranged into regions of differing depths.

Many objects are now becoming detached and independent entities that can be imitated, inserted in play routines, and related in space, time, and cause-and-effect sequences. They can also be studied, and their qualities fully explored from all aspects. Give your baby something you do not mind being ruined and watch him closely. He will probably vary what he does to the object to see how his actions affect it. Instead of just paying attention to his act of letting go, he now heeds the motion of his cup as it splatters to the floor. You rush to clean up the mess. Meantime, the baby studiously looks at it and tries to pick it up if you will let him. A grown-up's earliest memories may include a scene of himself as a toddler plopping an egg onto his grandmother's oriental rug, and the confusing hysteria of all the females in the household merely because he wanted to see what would happen to it when it fell.

A baby studies displacements very attentively, rolls a ball from the couch to the armchair, then back again; repeatedly stacks a series of rings on his stacking toy color cone; swipes his mother's jewelry box from her dresser, removes the bracelets, rings and earrings, then replaces them all as best he can; rotates and reverses his bottle and sets it by his plate on his feeding tray. He tries to accommodate features of unfamiliar objects instead of treating them as though they had all the properties of the nearest equivalent, familiar things.

He deliberately hides and finds his brother's coloring book

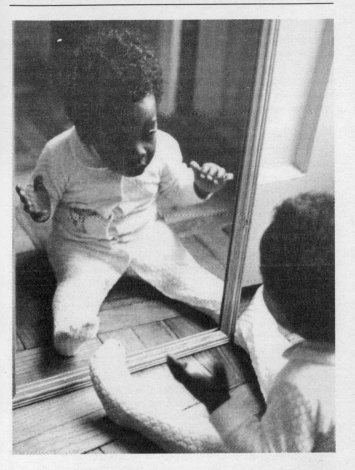

under the scatter rug, and removes an obstacle to reach for the toy he can see or even one he cannot. The baby begins to learn that just because his toy truck is not around, it has not vanished from the face of the earth. He discovers that the truck on the couch and the truck under the chair are the same, no matter where they are.

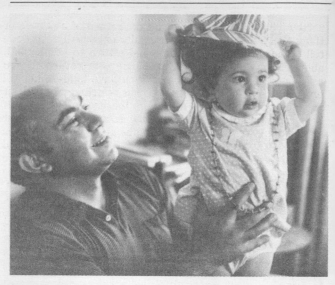

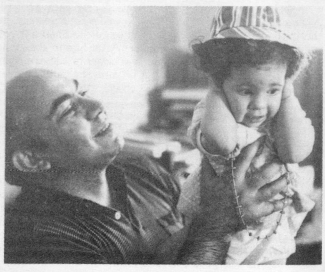

Now your baby can anticipate the return of a person or thing that he has released, manually or visually. You can tell because he is able to leave and return to you at will, allow you to leave him, and anticipate your return. If you ask your baby now to find a toy you have hidden, he will probably be able to find it if he has watched you hide it and you do not ask him to find it too long afterward. If he accidentally drops his toy behind an armchair, he might actually struggle to shove the chair away because he knows it's down there. His remembering, searching, and refusal to be diverted by other "finds" is the first step toward the more prolonged concentration of adults, and away from the distractibility characteristic of infancy and early childhood. In experiments at Harvard's Center for Cognitive Studies, Mrs. Judith Gardner found that young infants do not try to search for an object that they have watched disappear behind a screen. Somewhat older ones will visually track over the path the object followed before it disappeared. Only babies in the last several months of their first year begin to search beyond the disappearance point.

A baby's accomplishments in this department are still young. For example, if his ball rolls under an armchair, he hefts the chair away from the wall to get it. Should it roll under the love seat, which is too heavy for him to shove, he will give up after a few nudges and crawl to the armchair where he was more successful! A bit later, he will be clever enough to search *only* where the object was last seen.

Without this beginning concept of "object permanence," the baby would be very uncomfortable about rolling (dropping would be more accurate) a ball to his brother to throw back to him. As the baby plays with his brother, he *foresees* return of the ball he has thrown and is disappointed if his brother fails him.

Most wonderful of all, as the baby grows in his ability to distinguish people and things from their surroundings, he begins to sense that he himself is a person and an object among others. His whole body, as well as parts of it such as his hands and feet, is in space. *He* has his own texture, resistance, locomotive style, and he exists in relationship to other objects and people in his world.

THE TENTH MONTH

Motor Development	Language

Motor Development

Gross Motor

During this period there is a sequence of emerging motor skills: crawling, climbing, cruising, walking, etc.

Crawls on straightened limbs.

Stands with little support. May get self to stand independently by straightening limbs and pushing up and off from palms. Sidesteps along furniture.

Walks holding two hands. Climbs up and down from chairs.

Sitting

Sits down from standing. Gets onto stomach from sitting.

Can sit alone.

Fine Motor

Eight- to twelve-month-olds spend 20 percent of their waking hours actively exploring attributes of small objects by gumming (sucking), banging, striking, rubbing, turning around, and staring at them from different angles.

Carries two small objects in one hand. Dangles object from string.

Retrieval skills are mastered at this age; also taking things apart and trying to put them together.

Language

Vocalizing

Learns words and appropriate gestures, e.g., says "no" and shakes head; "bye-bye" and waves. May repeat word incessantly; make it a response to every question. May say one or two words besides "mama" and "dada."

Responding

Listens with interest to familiar words. Understands and obeys words and commands, e.g., "Give it to me, please."

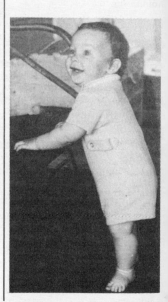

Please do not regard this chart as a rigid timetable. Babies are unpredictable. Some perform an activity earlier or later than the chart indicates.

Mental	Social

Mental

Sensory Response

Ranges distant space into regions of differing depths.

Sees individual objects as separate from others. Continues to learn about properties of objects; crumples paper, rattles box, listens to watch tick. Points, pokes, touches, and pries with extended index finger. Looks for contents of box. Grasps small objects in container. Looks at pellet if it drops out of container.

Eye-Hand Coordination

Reaches behind him for a toy without seeing it.

Memory

Searches for hidden object if he sees it hidden. Lifts inverted box or cup in search of toy. Searches briefly for object in second hiding place; if unsuccessful returns to first hiding place. Searches in same place for object he has seen hidden in various locations.

Body and Object Awareness

Increasingly imitates behaviors; rubs self with soap, feeds others.

Begins to sense he is an object among others. Begins to prefer one hand and side of body to the other. Points to body parts.

Discriminating and Associating

Tries out new acts for same goal; modifies old ones through trial and error.

Matches two blocks.

Social

Personal

Shows moods: looks hurt, sad, happy, uncomfortable, angry, and shows preferences; likes music, identifies body parts.

Imitates gestures, facial expressions, sounds. Begins sexual identity; e.g., boys begin identifying with males, girls with females. Grows aware of self, social approval and disapproval. May perform for audience at home; tries to win applause.

Interaction

More sensitive toward other children; cries if other child receives attention. Fears performing familiar activities; may regress to earlier stages.

Cultural Self-Help/Routines

Helps hold cup for drinking. Feeds self whole meals.

May have trouble sleeping.

Helps dress self. Pulls off hat for fun.

Small-muscle control of rectum.

Play and Playthings

Prefers one of several toys. Shows tenderness toward stuffed animal or doll. May sort his toys from others'.

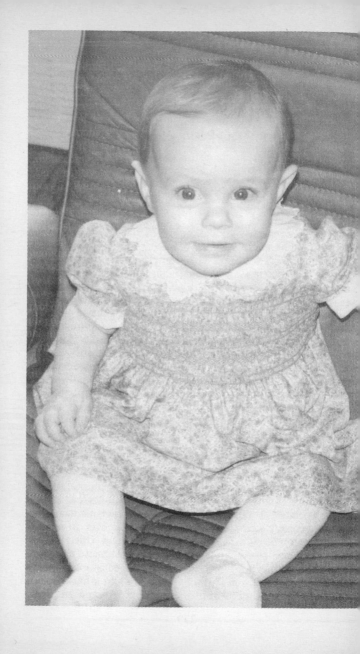

The Eleventh Month

A PROPER PERSON

During this month your baby is most likely to stand alone. His control of his upright body will improve as he gets used to being on his feet. He is becoming quite a handy little fellow. But as in the previous month, much of his energy and attention is turned to "social improvement," despite his extra dependence on you. He makes extensive use of imitation, his learning technique for discovering what people are all about. He grows more and more aware of approval and disapproval. Since being refused and limited, even "for your own good," is often hard for a baby to take, this can be a difficult time, especially when he is so engrossed in his preparations for walking.

Standing may become so important that your baby refuses to lie down. He stands next to furniture, he stands in the middle of the floor, he stands in his feeding chair, in his bath, as he is changed. He falls asleep standing in his crib. He stands for his examination by his pediatrician. Standing, he "helps" with his dressing. Holding onto your shoulders as you put on his overalls, he lifts one leg and then the other. Obediently he raises his arms so you can pull off his undershirt. Anything, as long as he is on his feet.

He becomes a public menace in his stroller. On the way to the grocery store, he stands and cranes over to snatch at passersby or claw at objects on the ground. Once inside, he stands and stretches for a large can of tomato sauce or a tantalizing bunch of grapes. Unless you constantly watch him, he is bound to fall. If you decide to find a harness for him, get one that gives him the freedom to stand and lean over, but prevents his tumbling out. But even if your baby is wearing a harness, he can pull his stroller over on top of himself unless it is solidly built.

His experimenting with standing may lead to other skills. As he topples forward, the momentum teaches him a new way to crawl. Arms and legs straightened out, bottom wagging left and right, he crawls on his "stilts" across the room. Climbing stairs is the next step, although coming down may not be so easy. You may find your baby partway up the stairs, pivoting around and ready to rocket into space, or perched precariously at the top of the staircase, on the verge of toppling down. Putting gates across the stairs will stop him for a while. One day, however, he may find the gate open and try to climb. Although a stair carpet will cushion a fall, the best safeguard in the long run is to try and teach your baby to climb in both directions. Although he may seem glued to his forward direction at first and unwilling or unable to try reverse, your persistence should pay off in his eventual understanding.

The baby may add other maneuvers to his standing ability, including squatting and stooping, just as he did when sitting, he will deliberately lean over and pick up a toy he has dropped. He squats, scoops the toy up in one hand, stands, then squats and scoops with the other. He is playing with the sensation of doing the same thing with different sides of his body. Then he stoops to collect his toy with *either* hand while he anchors himself with the free one at an armchair. These variations show the baby's increasing interest in depth and distance and his curiosity about how different maneuvers, such as dropping, will affect an object. Will it split, shatter, bounce, or clink when it hits? They also show his improving control of his body against gravity and illustrate his ability to use both hands simultaneously for different activities. The baby can hold a toy in one hand while pulling to stand with the other.

Your baby's manipulative behavior may be quite agile. Single-handedly he can carry his spoon to his mouth once you fill it for him. With both hands, he can hold his cup. Using one hand for picking up and eating bits of food and the other for complex maneuvers with the spoon is still a

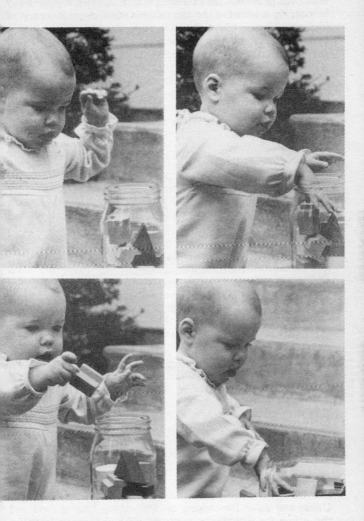

bit difficult. If he can pull off his socks and shirt, pull out shoelaces, and untie his own when asked, he is doing very well indeed.

If your baby seems anxious to walk, you may consider getting a walker for him. Before you do, try to imagine its potential effect on him—particularly if he is high-strung. Some babies react almost hysterically to the precocious mastery of a step and become too dependent on anything that helps with it. Dr. Brazelton writes about a baby boy who as soon as he was placed in a walker became a little wild

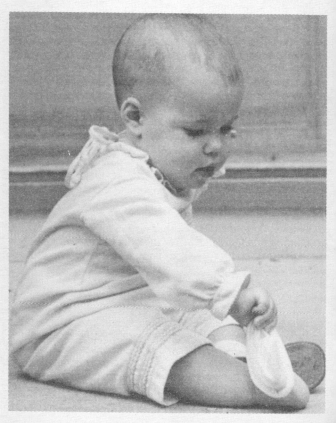

man, "losing contact with everything around him, propelling himself forward to the right, to the left, into furniture, bouncing over thresholds from one room to the other. No one could reach him, and he could not stop moving. When he was finally taken out, he screamed wildly as if separated from something desperately important to him." When he is ready, a baby commits all his pent-up energy to learning to walk. When he no longer has to learn for himself because he has a crutch, his own efforts may be checked and his unused energy makes him a very tense and unhappy person.

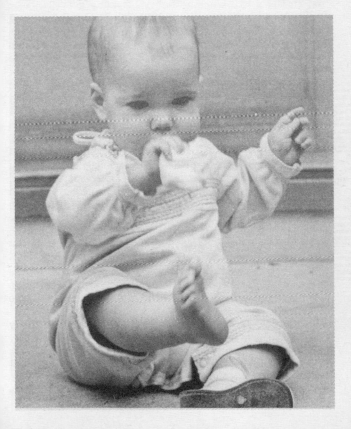

A baby enjoys his own experimentation much more. Some even discover their own crutch to walk with, often making themselves walkers from small chairs. Your baby, in leaning against a small chair, may make it move unexpectedly. Quite able to associate cause with effect now, he realizes that he has caused its motion. He pushes again and it slides again. If your baby happens to have selected your favorite Chippendale, turn another small chair on its back and let your baby practice with it. He may spend a fair portion of his day pushing and staggering along behind it. Besides being fun, this is a real teaching device. A baby gets the basic idea of walking by feeling and watching his weight shifting from foot to foot as he picks up each foot. Apparently babies have enjoyed this game for a long time. Many old wooden chairs are flattened on the backs of the posts from some baby's pushing on hard floors long ago.

Since babies are individuals, all eleven-month-olds do not perform the same miracles. Many are still not standing alone, while others are already walking by themselves. A very precocious baby will actually prefer to walk than crawl now. In contrast, a quiet baby is just standing supported. He may let his parents put him in a standing position, but he is clearly most excited when he laboriously hauls himself up. Unlike more active learners, he is slower but often more sure. He never tumbles backward from his new height, and when he comprehends the technique, he lets himself down gradually to sitting. Once he has mastered that hurdle, he feels less anxious about playing on his feet. If this sounds more like your baby, do not worry if some toddlers in the neighborhood seem more adept. Your baby's progress is average, not delayed. According to developmental norms based on studies of thousands of youngsters, the average age range for walking alone in the United States is twelve to fourteen months.

In addition, many quiet infants have a "flop-jointed" body type. They have rubbery, over-extensible joints that easily bend beyond a natural extended position and hardly seem to anchor anywhere at all. This kind of jointing makes locomotion harder, even when a baby wants to move. To give firmness to his joints when he stands and walks, the baby's musculature must be developed more than usual. So the child has to practice longer to gain the extra muscular strength he needs. Perhaps the quiet temperament that often accompanies the flop-jointed body type appropriately deters the inner-directed surge of physical activity until the body is able to handle it.

Many parents are concerned because their infants, when they start to stand, seem to have "rolled-in" or pronated feet. They balance with their legs apart on the inner edges of their feet and ankles rather than on the soles. As the baby's balance improves, he will no longer need this wide base of support. His feet and arches will strengthen and he will start "toeing in."

Some infants, however, toe in so much at the beginning that they occasionally stumble over their own feet. These babies should be left barefooted or given soft, flexible shoes, which are better for their feet and let their toes grip the ground. If your baby continues to have trouble, consult your pediatrician before he gets a bad feeling about walking. After your baby has walked for about a month, your pediatrician should evaluate his feet and legs anyway.

The right shoes are especially important. Shoes must fit perfectly and should not be too big to "allow for growth." Large shoes increase tripping and accentuate the way a baby walks, throwing his feet in or out to avoid the extra toe space.

More on Imitation

The imitation of the previous month is even more marked now. One of the basic requirements for the baby's imitative flair is the ability to remember behavior so that he can reproduce it. The baby must also have the ability to associate behavior and qualities with people and things. If your baby points upward when you say "airplane" or tries to meow when you show him a kitten, he is beginning to correctly associate certain qualities with their objects.

He will also play with differences. Dropping one object after another into a cup, he seems to hear the difference in the clunk of a block and the ring of a metal ball. If he tries the same thing with a glass, he will notice the new sounds the block and ball create against this new substance. When he tries to retrieve the objects from the glass, he first tries to reach them through its sides. Then he reaches into the open end. Although he has poured objects from a cup before, he has to relearn with a glass container because the visual cues from its transparent sides confuse him despite the familiar shapes and behavior. At first confounded because the total situation is different, the baby eventually breaks the whole scene into its component bits, learns to associate the containers despite their different materials, and later generalizes his new information about glass to other glass things.

A mirror is a bit trickier. Although he has learned to differentiate the mirror images of himself and his parents from reality, he may still reach for the reflection of a favorite toy. He may catch his mistake when he knocks his hand against the mirror.

Despite minor imperfections in technique, imitation proves more and more deliberate, sophisticated, and useful to the baby. He can cleverly reverse and adopt behavior he has watched. For example, your baby may hide a favorite toy of his brother's or sister's and laugh merrily when they find it. Since they have taught him the game with his toys and laughed at his discovery, he is a bit misled by their lack of amusement.

Through imitating, the baby also learns to talk and dress himself. From observing you dress him, he begins to help wiggle into clothes, pull off shirts when asked, stick his foot into a shoe, and figure out which leg or arm to extend. He tries to pull off his socks by catching the toe and pulling. But so far, he pulls backward and has little success unless the sock is practically off his foot anyway.

In learning to talk, a baby will copy his parents' inflections, as well as speech rhythms, and even produce facial attitudes in comically close mimicry. Your baby will try to approximate speech sounds, too. Though certain words are clearly familiar to him because he babbles back more when he hears them, his production of them lags behind his understanding. A few mumbled sequences may sound like *mama*, *dada, bye-bye, no-no,* but most of his speech is still gibberish.

During his prewalking stage, with all its exciting but frightening freedom, the baby is still very dependent on you. He identifies closely with your behavior and tries to imitate you at every turn. You may find him a constant attendant as he follows you about all day. If you wear a scarf on your hair as you work, he finds an old scarf to put on or wears the dust rag on his head. He begins to wipe the counter when you do, stir clumsily with a spoon as you are whipping up a cake, hang on heavily to the vacuum cleaner when you try to clean. He "goes and gets" simple objects for you and seems delighted when he returns with something you have asked for. He may even stand between your legs, leaning on them whenever you stop long enough, so that you have to step over him and may even trip on him during the day.

He watches you rock in a chair, crawls up into it, pushes you to get out, and begins to rock himself. He closes his eyes and hums just like mother when she is content. Although you probably rocked your baby when he was smaller, it now becomes novel, because the baby can do it for himself.

The baby's dependence on you is balanced by his increasing independence with his sibs and his attraction to his father. The baby will imitate the way his sibs play with toys, whack the floor with a toy hammer in delight, and jab at paper with a crayon as his sibs color. When his brother takes his hand to show him how to crayon, he pulls away and refuses to be shown. Even though he rejects the demonstration, his next efforts are closer to the scribbling motions his brother has tried to show him.

Almost all babies at this age are attached to their fathers and anticipate his homecoming at day's end. They act as if he behaves differently toward them and they are right. Fathers smile and talk less than mothers, but they are more interested in getting their babies actively involved in their physical environment. A baby boy especially enjoys "roughhousing" with father. Being bounced on daddy's foot, or thrown in the air, or picked up and spun around, jouncing on his back, or crawling all over him are great fun. The more violent the play, the better the baby likes it, as you can tell by his protests when father finally decides he wants to eat his dinner or read the newspaper. Some mothers see this turning to father as the baby's fatigue at being isolated with a female all day and as a desire for novelty. While this is partly true for all babies, father gives your baby boy an extension of his own active development, plus the chance to identify with another male. Just as a little girl is beginning to sense her femininity, the baby boy begins to realize some of his masculine identity.

No, No, a Thousand Times No

A baby this age is quite devoted to finding out about himself. As he stands and stoops, he is not just practicing physical skills. He is comparing the feeling of doing something with different sides of his body to see if there are various ways to achieve the same thing.

Another important part of a baby's identity is his ability to establish the meaning of no. Like standing, he must experiment with and practice it day and night. He will shake his head and say no to everything—even when he means yes. He loves the head movement and times his no so that it fits each swing. He is so taken with it, he may spend a whole meal flinging his head and refusing to eat. He refuses to cooperate during his bath—and catching his face to wash it as he swings his head is a real trick. He shakes his head through diaper changes and waggles his body in a total negative.

Along with a baby's ability to say no comes the realization of what the no of others means. Your baby will grow more aware of the difference between being good and being naughty. When he is "good," he constantly seeks your approval; for example, after he pulls on his sock or makes a block tower of two blocks, he calls out "See," with a grin that requests an approving comment. After he dutifully eats some of his lunch, he holds up the dish to be admired. When he finishes his bottle, he holds it out—shaking it to show how empty it is.

He is also conscious of the implications of his naughtiness. He learns to turn on the television. Frightened when it comes on with a blast, he scrambles to another room and waits for someone to turn down the volume. He learns rapidly that the sudden blare will bring someone. He has to be reminded repeatedly to leave it alone. Before he flushes the toilet in the bathroom, he pauses to look around hastily, then pulls the handle anyway. When his father comes to check his antics, he stands behind the bathroom door half-hidden and completely abashed.

When he is about to get into trouble, he looks at you as if to say, "Don't come after me," then scurries to his brother's toy chest (definitely off-limits), glances over his shoulder to check, lifts the lid, snatches a toy, and unwittingly lets the lid slam. He tucks the toy under his arm to conceal it, then crawls to a safe spot to enjoy himself. If you catch him at his play, his eyes widen and he smiles foolishly.

Clearly the baby knows what he is doing. He understands the meaning of no and some implications of his behavior. As

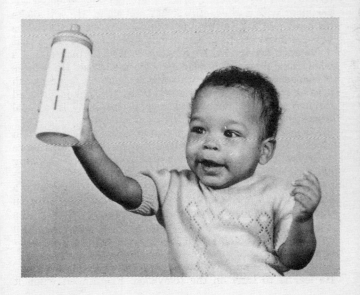

early as seven months of age, a baby can appear sheepish about being caught at something he is not supposed to do. Now he is a bit more aware of simple cause-and-effect actions. His repetition of your favorite swear word is breathlessly expectant because he is already aware of its specialness in *your* repertoire. You may find your baby's hearing ability gauged to his motivation and interest in performing what you request. Poor hearing can accompany things he does not want to hear, while he listens raptly to the ticking of his father's watch or your whispered "Want a cookie?" from across the room.

He is also becoming increasingly handy and mobile. Since he can move far and fast enough from you in a suddenly bigger and not always safe world, you must begin to set limits on his travels. Luckily, a baby's obedience and attachments to specific people develop at about the same time as his locomotion and comprehension of simple utterances. A baby at this age can understand his own no and simple commands so he can heed and comply with his mother's no-no and simple prohibitions. He is also able to understand more complicated demands, not necessarily because he comprehends the words being used, but because you amply cue him to your wishes by your facial expressions, tone of voice, and gestures. Some babies can also comply with known commands by stopping their own approach to a previously tabooed area or their reach for a forbidden object, mumbling "no-no" all the while or wagging their heads assertively as if to reinforce their own conviction. Such early self-control, by the way, has been experimentally associated with intelligence.

About the same time, your baby will try to test your no. When you are near, he may spend most of his time teasing you, pulling at your skirt, yanking at your shoes, banging your book. When you try to ignore him, he deliberately gets himself into spots where he needs help or goes for a no, such as an electric outlet, the TV, or the stove. If you do not object immediately, he may slow his pace and turn. When he sees you are watching, he smiles and continues full steam ahead. Usually, he is not even interested in the forbidden object per se because he rarely returns to it unless he has your attention. Often a child will try this game even when he has understood the rationale for the no and has accepted the prohibition.

Sometimes this testing is even more disturbing. At night, after he is in his crib, he will call you as many times as you will come. Mother or father will have to be firm or he will grow more and more demanding as the atmosphere tightens to the breaking point. Though still early, a few eleven-month-olds may begin consciously using tantrums as they recognize their power to control people in their world. When your baby wants a cookie that does not appear or a brother's toy that is off-limits, you may be stunned to see him drop dramatically to the floor, screeching and kicking in protest. Surprised and a bit overcome at his new "temper," you may at first give in rather than watch him scream. *Once is enough.* With that kind of encouragement, the baby will plummet into his routine every time he is refused something. Babies are quite clever about figuring out the appropriate behavior for the right person. If his regular sitter is singularly unimpressed, he will save his performance just for you.

Rather than punishing and confusing your baby, try to let him collapse and scream on the floor without responding. He will probably kick louder and roll his head even more at first. But if you persist long enough, he will probably quiet eventually—maybe with even a glance of surprise at you— and wordlessly resume his play. A calm end to such an episode is your sign that your baby is not in any real trouble. When a toddler has a real temper tantrum, he just cannot turn it off so easily.

The basic curbs to a baby's naughtiness are the same, though they may come from other family members too. Since you are not always speedy enough in removing the baby, an older child may learn to handle his no's himself. A sister's anger when the baby pulls over her doll table full of china may stop retrials permanently. Rather than anger, judiciously ignoring the baby's antics sometimes works. Often diversion is the answer. For example, when your eldest son drags the baby away from his toy chest by the legs, he only triggers another game. He pulls and baby waits until dumped across the room. Then he scrambles back. After all, brother means fun so far. But "No" and enticing the baby away with another toy works. Brother calls from another room or drags a toy before the baby's following nose, then quickly jumps to slam the lid on the toy chest. Your three-year-old learns what it takes many parents months to discover. Simply removing a baby from a goal without a change of interest only challenges him to repeat his original investigations more vigorously.

Sometimes you just have to say no forcefully. The baby may startle, turn to look at you to see if you mean it, pucker as if to cry, then finally pivot and go to something else. Although a few babies appear to know enough to stop themselves, most can get carried away and push their testing too far. Allowing anything as dangerous as a stove to be used to tease and involve you is foolish.

An experienced parent can be comfortable in a disciplinary role and not worry that the baby's feelings may be hurt by his or her sudden sharpness. A new mother and father, on the other hand, can feel very guilty when their baby looks wounded after they have taken a stand, although this does not negate its importance.

The best way to ensure a willingness to comply is not extensive training, discipline, or other massive attempts to modify the infant's natural course of development. It is a healthy, harmonious relationship between parent and baby. You can misuse the baby's attachment to you by curtailing his necessary explorations or you can use it positively, permitting him the freedom to grow and learn and limiting him only when he is in danger, or when you must for the sake of others in the family.

In a fascinating study, Dr. Mary D. Ainsworth of The Johns Hopkins University found that mother's discipline—the frequency of her commands and physical interventions—did not improve the baby's compliance with her commands. Quite the contrary, the more floor freedom she gave the baby, the more likely the baby was to control his own behavior. She found that certain motherly qualities—sensitivity to, acceptance of, and cooperation with the baby—were especially associated with the baby's obedience. Dr.

Ainsworth says, "The sensitive mother is aware of, accurately interprets and responds promptly and appropriately to the baby's signals and communications, and is able to see things from his point of view. The insensitive mother is geared almost exclusively to her own wishes, moods, and activity. Her interventions tend to be prompted by her own signals and so rarely relate to the baby's.

"The accepting mother accepts almost all aspects of the baby's behavior, including those things other mothers find hurtful or distasteful, and she also accepts the responsibility of caring for him without chafing at the temporary restriction of her usual activities. The rejecting mother may feel positively about her baby but is frequently overwhelmed by resentment and anger—which she may voice openly or display less overtly in her behavior toward him and her comments about him. The cooperative mother avoids imposing her will on the baby, and arranges the environment and her schedule to minimize any need to interrupt or to control him. When she intervenes she is adept at 'mood setting' which helps him to accept her wishes or controls as something congenial to him. At the other extreme, the interfering mother does not consider her baby as a separate person whose activities and wishes have a validity of their own. She seems to assume that she has a perfect right to do with him what she wishes, imposing her will on his, shaping him to her standards, and interrupting him arbitrarily without regard for his moods, wishes, or activity-in-progress."

Those mothers judged to be sensitive, accepting of the baby, and cooperative by these standards had babies who were naturally and willingly compliant to their commands. As Dr. Ainsworth points out, "The first and most important step in socializing a human being is a baby's willingness to do as he is asked. So the growth of an initial, unspecific disposition toward compliance may be critical for all later social development and learning."

THE ELEVENTH MONTH

Motor Development	Language
### Gross Motor	### Vocalizing
Some walk alone. Climbs chairs and tables.	Speech still primarily gibberish, with a few intelligible sounds.
Stands alone. Gets self to stand by straightening limbs and pushing up and off from palms, lifting trunk. May get self to stand by flexing knees, pushing off from squat. May stand against support and lean over.	Imitates inflections, speech rhythms, facial attitudes more accurately than speech sounds.
	Says two or three words besides "mama," "dada." Mumbles word or words for long periods.
Standing, may pivot body 90 degrees. Walks holding one or two hands. Climbs up stairs.	May use jargon; sentence of gibberish in which meaningful words are sometimes embedded. May express thoughts with single word.
### Sitting	
Squats and stoops.	### Responding
### Fine Motor	Begins to differentiate between words. Recognizes words as symbols for objects: "airplane," points to sky; "doggie," growls.
Interested in hinges and hinged objects; swings doors back and forth. Likes to turn pages of cardboard picture books.	
Holds crayons, makes marks. Grasps bell handle.	
May carry spoon to mouth.	
May use hands in sequence in feeding, or simultaneously, e.g., squat, pick up object in one hand, hold onto support with the other.	

Please do not regard this chart as a rigid timetable. Babies are unpredictable. Some perform an activity earlier or later than the chart indicates.

Mental	Social
### Eye-Hand Coordination	### Personal

Mental

Eye-Hand Coordination

Points at object through glass. May try to grab it through side of glass. Explores container-contained relationship. Fingers holes in a pegboard. Lifts lid from box. Unwraps cube. Pokes clapper of bell. Places and removes objects, such as a small block or spool into and from cup or box.

Memory

Increases imitation. Imitates scribble, ringing of bell.

Body and Object Awareness

Aware of his own actions and some of their implications. Compares same act done with each side of the body. May use both hands simultaneously for different functions.

Experiments with means to attain goal, e.g., uses small chair as a walker.

Discriminating and Associating

Associates properties with things; meows for kitten, points upward when he sees bird. May remove and place rings on a tower cone. May nest series of boxes. Turns pages of a book, not necessarily one at a time. Looks at pictures in book with interest.

Social

Personal

Reaches for mirror images of objects.

Asserts self among sibs.

Interaction

Increases dependence on mother. May infer some of mother's goals and her plans to achieve them. Begins trying to alter them through persuasion or protest.

Shows the beginning of social behavior by using objects.

Has established a strong relationship with primary caregiver. Relies on caretaker for feeding, reinforcement, a "job well done," and help when in tight spots.

Obeys commands. May inhibit his own behavior. Seeks approval. Tries to avoid disapproval.

Is not always cooperative. Refuses forceful teaching.

Establishes meaning of no. Shows guilt at wrongdoing. May tease and test parental limits.

Withdraws from strangers.

Cultural Self-Help/Routines

May pull off socks, untie shoelaces.

Play and Playthings

Imitates movement of adults and play of other children. Plays parallel to, not with another child. Protests curtailment of play. Extends but does not release toy to person. Opposes removal of toys.

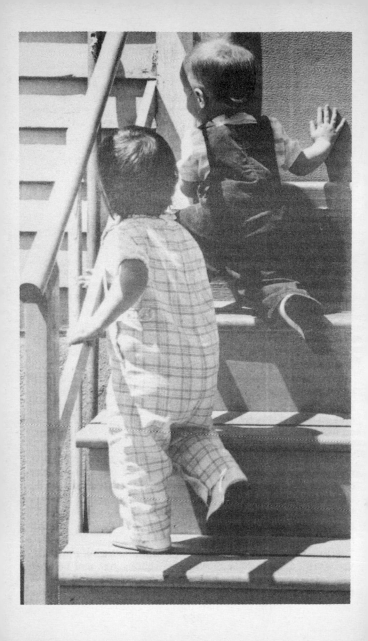

The Twelfth Month

STEPPING OUT

By the twelfth month, many babies are ready to walk. This
fascinating activity distracts the baby from what his parents
and most adults consider basics—eating and sleeping. But
there are even more profound consequences. The baby is
able to get to people and things and to explore space and
objects by himself in a way that will be far more efficient
than crawling. He is also more independent of adult control.
Yet fearful of this independence, he again grows anxious
about strangers and separations from you. Beyond this, the
balance between freedom and containment becomes an issue
that you and your baby must mutually solve.

Walking is the crowning achievement of this long and exciting "motor" year. The stepping reflex the baby had during
his first week of life and even more noticeably toward the
end of his first month may have allowed your baby to take
as many as fifteen consecutive steps across the floor as you
held him gently under the arms. For a long time this reflex
disappeared, only to surface again right after the middle of
the year, as the baby voluntarily stamped one foot or the
other and pumped his whole body up and down as you held
him under the arms. Later, when you held him by the hands,
he deliberately stepped in place and finally he took his first
steps with you. (Many babies are still at that point this
month or are just managing to stand alone.)

The first unsupported steps are often accidental. Perhaps
you let go of his hands as you are walking him and before
he quite realizes it, he has taken a step unassisted. Then
frustrated at being deserted, he flops to the floor. Some-

times it happens as a baby practices his standing maneuvers. Just as he did when he was perfecting his sitting skill, he twists the upper part of his body to reach for a toy behind him or to wave at you. At first he holds onto a prop to steady himself. Then he tries it without support. Soon he learns to balance as he turns by holding out *his* arms. Next, he pivots his *whole* body in sections—first the upper half, then the lower—by lurching around with arms carefully extended for balance. Believe it or not, these are the first unsupported steps.

Soon he applies the balance he has gained from turning. He spreads his wings, spinning his forearms and hands in tight flat circles for a kind of rotating propulsion. Straining every muscle, he begins to take steps from one to the other of you. He glues his eyes on his target, face drawn and intent, and totters forward on his toes. Squealing with joy, he collapses during his remaining steps toward waiting arms.

Within a week, he can navigate the expanse of an entire room. Arms high, with stiffened knees and a wide-legged gait, he swings his body sideways with each leg thrust. Like a bandy-legged old sailor, he clumps across the floor, sometimes losing his footing on the hardwood floor or a scatter rug. Cheerful about his downfalls, he simply gets himself together, pushes back to stand, and unless he stumbles again in the same spot, exuberantly shoves off again.

He learns how to slow down, catch himself, and turn around, and soon steers around edges and corners. Last of all, he learns to stop himself. Stopping in the middle of the floor is a real achievement. First stops are effected by falling or by clutching at passing people or furniture. When he finally can halt at will, he practices it constantly.

In a matter of a week, he changes from a person who looks as if he wants to but does not dare to one who can not get enough. Parental praise and enthusiasm can noticeably lengthen the stretches of steps he takes before tripping. With or without you, he staggers, topples, halts, but always starts forward again hour after hour. You may be fascinated with your baby's tireless, almost feverish devotion. The exuberance and accomplishment radiating from your baby's face show his recognition that he has attained another major

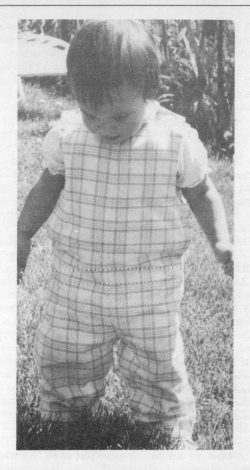

goal. Babies are so consumed by their own walking prowess that they will actually swagger off the top of a table from which they have cautiously crawled only a few months before.

His determination when he first walks affords a precious glimpse of the inner force that pushes young animals from one level of development to the next and drives them to conquer their environments. His feelings also testify to the joy and pride that come from doing something by oneself.

Walking will be an unwieldy accomplishment for a long time. It definitely should not be considered a performance for others, particularly people the baby considers strangers, in a strange place. It still demands the infant's total concentration. Crawling is baby's business approach to his environment, the one he uses when he really wants to go places fast or freely explore strange scenery. Just as you could tell around the half-year mark how new the baby's sitting skill was by the height of his arms, you can gauge his prowess in walking by whether or not he needs to extend his arms high. As his walking balance improves, he will gradually lower his arms. This important step means that a baby has learned to balance himself from within his body, by controlling the muscles of his trunk. Then he can master other maneuvers, such as using his hands while he walks. The first such actions are usually in rhythm with the legs' motion because they can be assimilated better into the total body action. Partly for this reason, partly because it is so social, one of the first additions to walking is waving and saying "bye-bye." The baby learns to flap his hand as you leave the room.

Those babies who have been walking for a couple of months may be adding more complicated maneuvers. Yours may balance his toys as he walks. Much like an older child walking on a fence, he holds his full hands high. Or he may walk backward, pulling a toy so he can watch it as he pulls (even though he backs right into furniture). Walking backward is easier for your baby than you might guess—creeping and crawling, after all, began backward.

For most babies, walking is a rather rigid task. The baby is not at ease enough yet to take pieces of the whole performance and translate them readily to other physical skills. Pushing himself in a kiddy car, for example, which also requires alternating use of the legs, takes many weeks to learn. He may inch along tagging after a brother and sister on their tricycles. First he will push with both feet, sometimes with one at a time, then both again laboriously. Alternating the feet to push is just different enough from alternating them to walk to cause difficulty. The baby has to balance seated instead of upright and he must also push back against the ground, as well as down. Recognizing the rigidity with which infants learn many skills, Dr. Myrtle McGraw, a leader in infant research for almost four decades, has actually taught roller-skating to babies. She trains them *after* they have learned to balance upright, but *before* they have locked into a specific way to displace their body weight forward.

Walking has a curious companion. Just as it appears, swimming behavior begins to show in the tub. Like walking, swimming goes through three phases. Newborns have a reflex ability to swim. They can squiggle through the water quite competently. Then for a long stretch after their third month, they have trouble in the water. Now if you support your baby gently under the chest, his body will undulate, his arms will circle naturally at his sides, and his legs will kick alternately. These swimming movements are inherited from our amphibious ancestors. Infants are naturally beguiled by water and love swimming. They will swagger in over their heads unless carefully watched. Fear of water and of getting one's head under the surface comes in the second or third year because of greater awareness of what water can do. Before this fear develops, teaching an infant to swim is quite easy. Unless swimming is continued regularly from this time on, however, these movements will be abandoned as sensory experience and judgment expand.

Language Learning

By the first birthday, most infants clearly understand many words and phrases. They may obey simple commands to *bring* or *give*, and so on. Most may be able to point to a familiar object in a picture book. The absence of expressive jargoning and failure to understand any beginning words or phrases call for a professional checkup of the child's hearing.

THE ANATOMY OF BEGINNING SPEECH

The shape of a baby's sound-making organs change. For example, the vocal chords grow, and the distance from the glottis to the lips lengthens; the roof of the mouth arches differently. Lack of teeth and tongue control probably impedes the articulation of certain sounds, for instance, *t* and *s*. The infant's neck also lengthens, and the jaws widen and lengthen. Gradually the maturing of the vocal apparatus permits the production of recognizable vowel and then consonant sounds.

Besides rather awkward individual articulation, the speech organs are also a bit uncoordinated. The production of every speech sound requires an appropriate signal from the brain to each of more than a hundred muscles in the

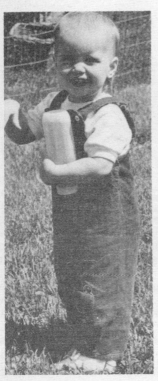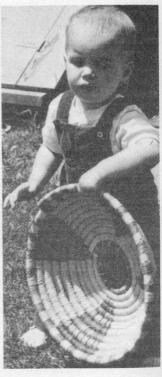

tongue, lips, cheeks, palate, jaws, larynx, diaphragm, and thoracic and abdominal walls. With the organs of speech growing at different rates and the brain itself slowly changing, small wonder that the smooth meshing of speech mechanics takes time.

The most important developments of the first year of language acquisition are mental, and a baby's word productions generally lag behind his capacity to understand the language.

Handy Helper

Walking, the most visible and dramatic physical achievement, tends to mask other exciting physical happenings of this period in your baby's life. As you may have noticed to your amusement and dismay, your baby is becoming more and more handy even though he still cannot handle many things well. Try to offer him a bowl and watch his "overlap grasp" as he takes it from you. Until he is about eighteen months old, he will place his fingers on the inside of the bowl, his thumb on the outside, and the rim in the palm.

Still, he has come a long way. One reason is that some of the bones of his hand and wrist are now firm. Instead of the soft cartilage of early infancy, the baby has more to work with. From the visibly labored eye-hand coordination he achieved in grasping at six months, he can now reach for something while looking the other way. From crude, raking motions with a clawlike hand, he comes to handle small items neatly with thumb and forefinger. From total involvement of his whole body, he has refined and limited his efforts to his arm and hand muscles. From the two-handed reach of midyear, he now offers a preferred hand along the line of sight.

Your baby, like most his age, is probably using the right hand as the active explorer and the left as a container and holder. At about four and a half months of age, many infants use both hands equally. Now about 70 percent of them will accept a proffered object with the right hand. You will also see this preference in finger-feeding, in reaching, and in thumb-sucking. At Harvard's Center for Cognitive Studies, visiting infants show their end-of-year dexterity by pushing up and holding a sliding, see-through trap door with one hand and reaching inside for a toy with the other. A more precocious baby can rest his chin on his left hand while leaning on his left elbow and maneuver his push toys with his right hand.

Some babies now can hold onto more than a couple of things at a time. As you may recall, your baby at about seven months dropped a toy he was holding to take your offering—as long as you caught him before his toy was on its way to his mouth. Possibly at about ten months, he took the second toy in his free hand without dropping the first. If you offered a third plaything, one of the others had to go as he took the new one. Now if you offer him that third toy, he may put one of the first two in the crook of the opposite arm and take the new object with his free hand. As long as his arm holds out, he will continue to accept toys. He is becoming a competent tool user, just like other humans and very unlike most animals. By using his arms and hands as holders and movers, he is converting features of his world into means of attaining goals of his own choosing—in this instance, getting toys without using parent to do it for him. With this new confidence in his hands, he will become more and more free to use them for truly new methods of getting things done just for the fun of it.

With all these skills, some active twelve-month-olds can undress themselves completely whether you want them to or not. Your baby may untie his shoelaces, slip off his shoes and socks, or go the whole route, slip off overalls and diapers, and lurch out of the house. Reversing the overalls so the zipper or buttons are in back will avert this minor "disaster." One morning you may find your baby naked in bed, his clothes cast overboard. Perhaps because of your initial rewarding reaction, he may take off as many clothes as he can manage every nap and night. When he has had a bowel movement, the crib, of course, is a wreck. Sleepers with snappers in the back that are pinned securely or a sleeping bag with the zipper in the back will block his agile little hands.

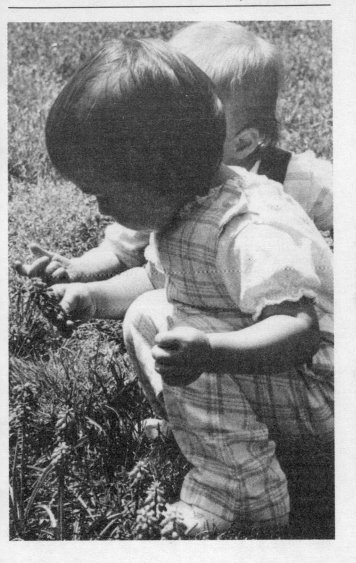

Food? Forget It!

As you have probably learned over the past year, a major
step such as walking has far-reaching implications for you.
The baby's fervor and single-minded dedication to walking
will interfere with his eating and sleeping. His awareness
that walking is another means of bringing about separation
from you will bring on a temporary period of fearfulness.

All this activity means the slowing of your baby's weight
gain, even if he remains a good eater and enjoys every
mouthful. Weight gain first slackens off for most babies by
seven months, when they are crawling and losing interest
in food. Now even more calories are burned as fuel for the
baby's constant activity. Possibly his body is able to use less
of what he eats because finger foods are not as thoroughly
chewed and digested as mashed baby foods. Even so, your
baby can absorb what he needs from a lumpy diet. The
slowing of weight gain is good despite the once-popular belief that healthy babies are fat babies. At this stage your
baby should be developing muscle tissue, not fat.

The independence that walking inspires may further com-
plicate meals and vex parents. In fact, the baby may begin
to use food against you, much like his new no's and even
tantrums, as one aspect of his self-differentiating and assertion over his environment. So forget your dreams of a three-

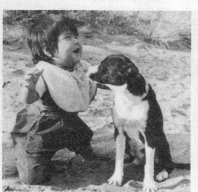
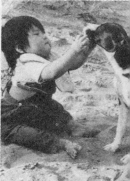

meal-a-day, well-balanced diet for your baby. Do not be surprised if he eats one good meal, one so-so meal, and rejects another. He may have very definite likes and dislikes, refuse to try new foods, stick to only three or four favorites, and insist on feeding himself. You may lament all this, but trying to convert him to a well-rounded diet would be more trouble than it is worth. One good meal and four "acceptable" foods are par for the course for babies this age. Babies who comply with their mothers' notions of "a proper diet" are rarities. You will do a good job just sticking to the basic food requirements.

If you are still worried that the baby's new idiosyncracies will mean lower intake of essential foods, some pediatricians suggest waiting to wean him to the cup. Keeping the baby on the bottle allows him to meet his daily milk requirement of one pint since it provides a known quantity of milk. Having two ways to give him milk is also an asset if he is still unpredictable about using a cup. If a bottle interferes with his appetite because his anticipation of it at a meal's end distracts him from solids, cut him down to two bottles of eight ounces each, and give them long enough after meals so the baby disassociates them. Knowing his needs are satisfied will allow you to relax and not push your baby to eat. Without pressure from you, he should not be a feeding problem by age three or so.

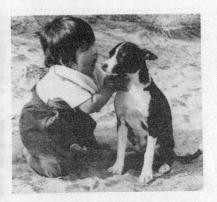

In fact, you should no longer be participating in his feedings at all. Many babies at this age interpret parental participation as pressure and use it to key off a negative reaction to the whole meal. You might consider serving finger foods and leave choices to the child. In a now-famous experiment by Dr. Clara Davis, one-year-old babies who were allowed to choose freely from a buffet of wholesome foods, with no adult pressure, selected and ate what they required and rounded out their own diets over a month's time.

Some babies, however, still want an intimate give-and-take with mother. As long as your baby wants to be fed, feed him. Even babies who can hold their bottles and wield their own cups perfectly well may refuse to do so. Your baby may willingly accept utensils as playthings at mealtime and drink from a cup when you hold it for him, but wag his head emphatically and clench his hands when you try to place them around it—almost as if he feels that feeding him is still your job, which he is not going to assume. He may sense that as soon as he holds his own bottle and manipulates his cup or spoon he can be left alone with them, and he still prefers having you at hand.

Sleep? What's That?

Walking and the discoveries it allows may also mean increased resistance to bedtime. The baby cannot quiet down when he is supposed to sleep and he wakes easily. For many babies, rocking on hands and knees and rolling and banging their heads, like thumb-sucking, accompany gushes of physical growth. The leftover energy from the day's adventures must be expended in some way, either when the baby tries to sleep or wakes up to semiconsciousness. Rocking on his hands and knees, your baby may soon learn he can jounce his crib across the room to the wall, squeaking and banging against it alternately. Before he becomes used to the noises, it might be well to grease and tighten the screws of his crib.

Unless upsetting to other family members, these outlets should not be restricted. Thick rugs or rubber casters under the crib posts will help stop the sound from carrying. Harnesses or other restraints, on the other hand, counteract the infant's natural urge to move and may make him hit his head more violently. The best way to help the baby is an after-dark session of crooning and gentle rocking as you feed him his last bottle. Although it may take as much as half an hour from your evening, feeling his tense little body begin to relax will be worth the time. Not only do you help the baby directly, you also set a valuable pattern for the future that he may include in his own repertoire. Being able to break from intense activity to relaxation is a must for many hardworking, driving adults.

The baby may also have trouble napping. After they learn to walk, babies are ready for one nap that fits into a daily pattern harmonious with the schedule of the rest of the family. Different infants have different cycles in this respect. But some babies, strange as it seems, are ready to nap in the morning soon after the night's long sleep. A morning nap, however, tends to make a baby fussy by midafternoon and too tired to eat his supper. A short collapse about 5:00 P.M. only refuels him for a long evening, and bedtime gets later and later. If your baby prefers a morning nap, you might begin delaying it until 11:00 A.M., then feed him a small lunch and put him down for two hours. When he wakes, feed him a second lunch, which will tide him over to an early supper. When he can last, feed him later, and gradually introduce him to a noon lunch and an early afternoon nap. This slow, steady pressure, an excellent way to adjust a baby's day, frees the evening for a needed respite from the baby, much as you love him.

Fearful Again

Coincident with rapidly increasing locomotion is a third phase of dependence on mother and fear of strange people and situations. The first usually occurs at four or five months, with the thrust of visual development, and the second at around eight months, when the baby can get about on the ground. Through with the frustration and emotional buildup before walking, the baby senses some of the consequences of being mobile. Just as he would insist on your pulling him up when he was learning to stand, now he will only walk holding onto your hands, and will totter only toward the arms of the people he trusts the most. He rightly distrusts his unpredictable sister, who is too easily diverted by any toy in her vicinity to catch him if he should topple. He may cling to you often, scamper after you when you leave a room, plead to be picked up, fuss in the evenings until you cuddle him, cry easily, and curl up in your arms when a new friend visits.

Many toddlers this age will still socialize with strangers in their own homes. Your baby may display his interest in socializing by fiercely hugging visiting toddlers, pressing them down when they try to stand, showing off his toys, and even permitting them to play with a few. But in the park, or yard, or during visits, he may clasp you tightly and refuse to join other youngsters.

Because of this intensified dependency, any separation from you, such as moving, hospitalization, or your long-awaited vacation will be particularly hard on your baby. If you must leave him, choose a caretaker such as a grandparent whom he knows, and who knows him, who understands and accommodates to his ways. If he has a brother or sister, leave the sibling with the baby for comfort and company. In his own home, with his own routines, the loss will be easier for him to bear and the baby will cope with the new situation a little better. Caring for him will be easier, too.

While you are away, the baby may regress to an earlier stage of behavior. Many babies do this when they need to apply their energies to emotional adjustment. He may stop walking altogether, and his general progress may slacken, or he may be almost "too good." Even though he appears to have done well with familiar grandparents or a pleasant nurse, you should expect a reaction either immediately or soon after you return. You may find a very sober or a very aggressive baby. Once secure, he may kick the nurse about whom he could not dare reveal any bad feelings when he had only her to count on. He may be more clinging, cranky, anxious about your whereabouts, and more fearful of strangers than usual even for this time of heightened dependence, or he may need to get back at you for your desertion.

If you can handle your baby's "retribution," expressing his resentment will be good for him. Still noticeably wary about your whereabouts, he will eventually resume walking, but not until you have been back awhile will he assume his usual spirit.

Disapproval from family or friends sways many parents from their instinctive responses to their babies' pleas for extra support and physical contact. Try to remember that people have many reasons for doing things. Your spouse's friend may accuse you of spoiling the baby when you are not. Perhaps he envies the baby's ability to regress to an earlier dependency that he as an adult cannot assume. Perhaps an unmarried sister wishes that the baby might turn to her. Other members of the family may resent the baby's ability to monopolize your attention. Certainly the baby's brothers and sisters envy his ability to get what they are now too "grown-up" to ask for. Remember, too, that the baby is yours and your spouse's. You understand him and your feelings best, so you are the best judges of your baby's needs. Even though you yourself might worry about spoiling him, *you* know down deep whether or not he has special needs at this time. This phase is common to babies in most of the world. It will pass once the baby is used to his new ability to separate from you and is able to incorporate it into his style of response. When he learns to do something about your absence, his anxiety will ebb. With support, your baby can reconsolidate his emotional resources to move toward greater autonomy.

One last thing to keep in mind is that babies who are unattached to their parents are rarely very dependent on them. It is a compliment to you and your nurturing that the baby trusts and cares for you.

Not only do babies with parents sensitive and responsive to their needs and aware of their unique personalities have a physical, pleasurable, and comforting relationship with them, they also seem to be ahead in intellectual areas. They are much more able to conceptualize inanimate objects and people as permanent—a vital mental skill—with stable shapes and qualities whether or not they are out of sight and beyond contact.

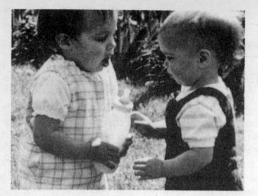

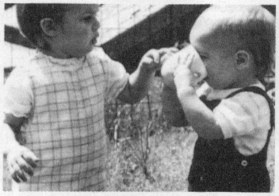

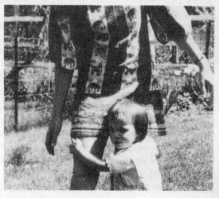

Limits—Personal and Otherwise

The baby's fearfulness, which is limited to strange places and people, does not, of course, limit his explorations at home. His new physical and social freedom means that you must strike a balance between too much containment, which becomes oppression for the baby, and too much liberty, which can mean discomfort for the rest of the family or danger for the baby. Older children do need times when they are not saddled with the baby's constant presence and even parents need some relief now and then.

The whole issue of containment, physical or social, is difficult for a baby and his parents. Discipline is all the harder now because the baby needs to exercise his brand-new "self-ness" and because he *is* more privileged. His daily "firsts" and accomplishments are toted out proudly.

Anger and discipline are often tough issues for parents to face honestly, especially if they have troubled memories of their own childhoods. Most adult responses, especially anger, are completely ineffective during a child's temper tantrum. Frequent discipline for errors can yield a sense of powerlessness that effectively stops learning. Your baby can understand an honest outbreak of anger if you follow it by holding him and explaining that you are sorry about your anger but you felt it was right, more easily than smoldering

Independence-Dependence

Forcing independence is not the same as encouraging it. Providing an infant with a task that is too difficult at the time will only frustrate him and elicit dependency responses. When your baby shows signs of readiness, presenting him with suitable challenges will further his development. Although six-month and older infants appear to demand less and desire to do increasingly more on their own, parents need always to be aware that the push toward independence is a slow, arduous, and long process. Self-reliance can be fostered but never rushed. One cannot "train" for independence.

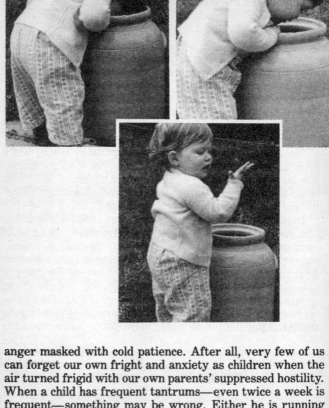

anger masked with cold patience. After all, very few of us can forget our own fright and anxiety as children when the air turned frigid with our own parents' suppressed hostility. When a child has frequent tantrums—even twice a week is frequent—something may be wrong. Either he is running into a wall of "don'ts" or he has found that he can manipulate his parents. Sometimes the situation seems to involve no one but the baby. His budding attempts to sort "yes" from "no," "do" from "don't," "out" from "in," "down" from "up" create inner turmoil in him, too. Some babies have such a hard time with these decisions, especially when they are tired, that any mild rebuke or refusal may unleash a tempest of unapproachable screaming, head-banging, and kicking. Reaching a child in the midst of a tantrum is very difficult.

Perhaps tantrums recall our own painful memories of ambivalence or impotence in making critical decisions. Screaming, slapping, or spanking the toddler are selfish ways to rid ourselves of our own bewilderment and tensions. They do not help the child. Waiting until your baby's hysteria has calmed and then comforting him with understanding and love are far better. While you are waiting, you can do a little self-examination to see what caused the tantrum and whether it could have been avoided. These responses are a distinct improvement over giving in to the baby's demands because you are afraid of his temper. Although it may not be apparent to you at first, your firmness will help the baby find his own personal controls and ultimately cut through the very indecision that drives him wild now. Developing these personal limits is crucial to your baby as he learns to move through the inner world of thought and feeling, just as recognition of physical limitations is necessary for learning to navigate the world of space and objects.

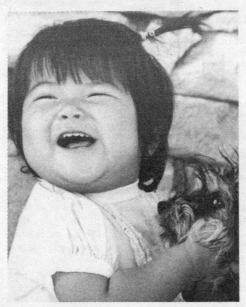

THE TWELFTH MONTH

Motor Development	Language
### Gross Motor	### Vocalizing

THE TWELFTH MONTH

Motor Development

Gross Motor

A "cruiser," carefully moving about while holding onto an object or person for support.

Walks when supported. Can pull self up to standing position.

Steps off low object. Many twelve-month-olds begin walking without support, but are still clumsy at running and climbing. All require watching.

Gets self to stand by flexing knees, pushing off from squat. Standing, pivots body 90 degrees.

Walks, but still prefers crawling. May add maneuvers to walking, e.g., stopping, waving, backing, carrying toys.

Climbs up and down stairs. May climb out of crib or playpen. Makes swimming movements in tub.

Sitting

Can ascend an upholstered footstool.

Lowers self to sit gracefully.

Fine Motor

Thumb apposition complete.

Takes covers off containers. Prefers one hand. Holds with one, maneuvers with the other.

Can point with index finger. May push objects.

Language

Vocalizing

Controls intonation patterns. Produces more sounds specific to native language of parents.

Aware of expressive function of language (e.g., repeats "damn" expectantly).

Practices words he knows. Besides "mama," "dada," says two to eight words: possibly "no," "baby," "bye-bye," "hi"; words that imitate sound of object, e.g., "bow-wow."

Babbles short "sentences."

Responding

Words begin to assist in discrimination of object classes; "pei" is airplane and kite, i.e., flying objects.

Mental	Social

Mental

Eye-Hand Coordination

Reaches accurately for something as he looks away.

Perceives objects as detached and separate, to be imitated, inserted into play routines, and related in time and space. Studies displacements of objects; rotates, reverses, and stacks things; places and removes them in and from containers, e.g., puts three or more blocks in cup; takes blocks and pellets out of box. Unwraps toys.

Memory

Finds toy under box, cup, pillow. Searches for hidden object even if he hasn't seen it hidden, but remembers where object was last seen. If toy is hidden in a second place, may search for it there.

Remembers events for longer and longer time.

Imitates a model more deliberately and precisely. Imitates behavior of an absent model.

Body and Object Awareness

Senses self as distinct from other things. Uses and reaches with a preferred hand. Uses one hand as holder, the other as explorer. Through active trial and error, may find effective ways, truly new to him, to solve problems.

Social

Personal

Expresses many emotions and recognizes them in others.

Distinguishes self from others.

Interaction

Fears strange people and places. Reacts sharply to separation from mother. Definitely prefers certain people to others.

To counter abusive behavior of older siblings, one-year-olds learn how to complain and use parents to defend their rights.

Develops sense of humor.

Gives affection to humans and objects such as toys and clothes. Negativism increases.

Mimics action of others. Intently watches people and their activities.

Cultural Self-Help/Routines

Refuses eating a meal, new foods, mother's feeding; resists napping; may have tantrums.

Usually insists on self-feeding. Takes three meals a day. Holds cup to drink. Uses spoon. Plays with saucer.

May undress self. Cooperates in dressing. May have trouble sleeping; one afternoon nap.

(continued)

Motor Development	Language

Please do not regard this chart as a rigid timetable. Babies are unpredictable. Some perform an activity earlier or later than the chart indicates.

Mental	Social

Discriminating and Associating

Differentiates personalities; trusts differentially.

Builds tower of two or three blocks after demonstration. Can group a few objects by shape and color. Likely to put one of two objects in mouth, another under arm, grasp a third. May mentally process actions or events before acting them out.

Play and Playthings

Plays simple games with understanding. May give up toys upon request.

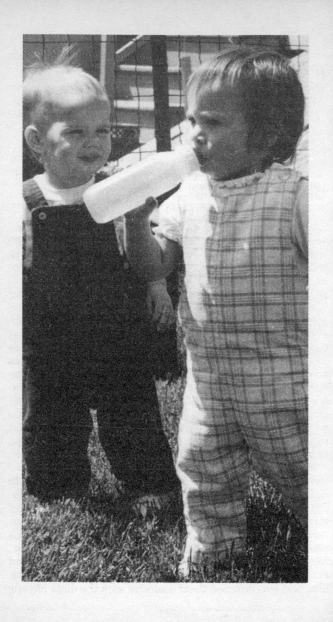

Epilogue

Looking Back

It's been a long and exciting year, hasn't it? When you and your baby began your life together twelve months ago, you were strangely new to each other. He was so very weak and helpless. All he could do was lie down. If you tried to sit him up, his gigantic head (with its "dangerous" soft spot) flopped every which way—so much so, you sometimes thought it might snap off his tender neck. If you touched him in certain spots, you triggered reflexes that came from every level of the evolutionary scale. The squeaks that emerged were unlike those of any language you had ever heard. He even looked funny. His skin was as wrinkled as an old man's, and he looked blue and waterlogged. But the nurse kept telling you that this was *your* baby. Your pediatrician repeatedly assured you that all those weird twitches and spasms were perfectly normal and had nothing to do with bad genes inherited from your great aunt on your mother's side or the caudal anesthetic you took in your last hour of delivery.

After you won your first terrifying struggle to get your newborn to take the nipple and "please eat," he began to demand so much of you, you thought you'd weep from fatigue, and sometimes you really did. He ate and ate and ate. If you were a few minutes late, his piercing, insistent screams were enough to shatter your skull. The worst of it was that hunger, your first "explanation" for everything, wasn't always the problem. How desperately your mind raced over the countless details that could be wrong with him, and you matched them uselessly with the dicta of your

381

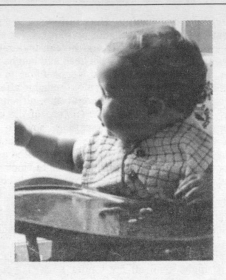

mother and that bright young nurse from the hospital's mini-course on baby care. It took you weeks to realize that you had come up with your own solutions, that sometimes your baby cried because he was as frustrated as you were with his inability to reach out and get into that world that was going on above his prone and clumsy little body.

All that you *were* sure of was that ferociously strong, somehow reassuring grip on your finger from an incredibly tiny fist; the jerky, valiant efforts of a wobbling head to turn toward you; and the intense, momentary gaze from eyes still bruised from the battle of birth and its aftermath. Even then, how could you be certain of anything in the hospital when you had him only those precious few minutes after feedings? Still, he seemed to be picking up some echoes from an environment totally alien to the warm, safe womb he had been at home in. These things (not the "love" the baby books preached) guided you and so did your sense that somehow you mattered to him and you had to help because no one else cared as much.

And here he is now, just a year later. He can sit any-where, stand, stoop, climb, and probably walk. Next thing you know, he'll be running. He can reach out for things, grab them with a favorite hand, and search for something lost. He can say a few words and he can understand you! He smiles at you, throws back his head and laughs with you, hugs you, gets angry at you, and weeps if you go away. He is such a lovable creature he even extends his affection to a brother or sister and to his grandparents, although he can be pretty cool toward strangers. Instead of the chaos of 3 A.M. feedings and inexplicable crying, now he eats and sleeps at pretty much the same times you do. What is more, he likes it that way. He relishes certain tastes and smells and detests others. He wants to listen to, look into, and manipulate *everything*. He can attend closely to a block tower he is building *and* listen carefully for the sounds at the front door signaling father's homecoming! He can deliberately empty all your pots and pans from the kitchen cabinets merely to solve the problem of how to get them all back in again. Though such relentless curiosity can be totally exasperating at times, his sheer, exuberant joy in learning and discovering as simple a thing as his face in a mirror delights you and your spouse constantly. Most of all, he has become a person among others. He is somewhat aware of this too, because he can remember people, places, events, and things, and he senses that they have substance independent of his.

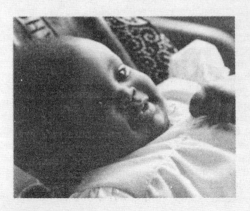

Can you believe it? You have come so far together in such a short, whirlwind time. He was born only a breath ago. Together you have learned to navigate the worlds of people, space, and thought. Now that he has begun to get around physically, your toddler will practice upright balancing and master the techniques of handling himself physically in more and more situations. His world, enlarged beyond mother and father, requires communication with people less tuned in to his signals and silent cues. So he has a purpose and readiness for mastering words and learning the grammar of his language. Having begun a career of reciprocation and exchange with you and the immediate family, your child is ready to use his language, his culture, and his mind to chart his own special course in the world beyond infancy.

Looking Ahead

If you enjoyed using this book to follow the month-by-month development of your child, you will find *The Second Twelve Months of Life* equally helpful (New York: Bantam Books, 1980).

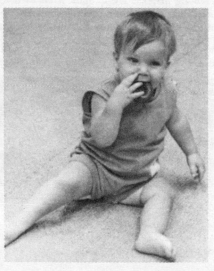

Your child's second year is also a period of tremendous potential. It is during these months that great strides are made in language acquisition and learning, in the development of self-confidence and ego, and in adjustment to the "outside" world.

The Second Twelve Months of Life is an invaluable guide to this vital period. It offers a diversity of approaches to child-rearing, as well as the "ages and stages" insights of professionals. It helps you recognize your child's drive for independence, sources of fears and anxieties, and the shaping of personality and habits. It analyzes month-by-month growth and provides monthly progress charts.

As a bonus, there is included a 39-page mini child-development course that you will find indispensable in preparing yourself and your child for new situations and encounters in the second year.

(If your bookstore does not carry it, ask them to order it from Bantam Books, 1540 Broadway, New York, NY 10036.)

Some Books For Parents

Baby and Child Care, by Benjamin Spock (New York: Pocket Books, 1992) continues to be the popular standard reference for health and child-development problems of infants and preschoolers.

Caring for Your Baby and Young Child, by Steven P. Shelov (New York: Bantam Books, 1991) has practical advice under the seal of the American Academy of Pediatrics.

Child Health Encyclopedia, by Boston Children's Medical Center Staff and Richard I. Feinbloom, M.D. (New York: Delacorte Press, 1975), is the most complete guide to child health and the diseases affecting children. For the first time, eighty medical experts share their knowledge and insights with parents. Written in nontechnical language. A must for every home!

The First Twelve Months of Life Companion, by Theresa Caplan (New York: Perigee Books, 1992) is an attractive, up-to-date record-keeping book.

Infants and Mothers: Differences in Development, by T. Berry Brazelton, M.D. (New York: Delacorte Press, 1983), is an authoritative guide for new parents. Reviews the health habits and emotional development of an active, passive, and "normal" infant in the first twelve months of life.

The Magic Years, by Selma Fraiberg (New York: Scribners, 1968). A very popular, useful discussion of how children mature from birth to six years of age.

Mother's Almanac, revised edition, by Marguerite Kelly and Ella Parsons (New York: Doubleday, 1992), is one of the first comprehensive books on child care from the point of view of mothers who are writers. A witty and reassuring book.

Pregnancy, Birth and the Newborn Baby, by The Boston Children's Medical Center (New York: Delacorte Press, 1976), is an up-to-date compendium by nine authors, all specialists in medicine, psychology, or anthropology. It is extraordinary because it presents, without bias, available birth and parenting alternatives.

Feed Me, I'm Yours, by Vicki Lansky (New York: Bantam Books, 1981), presents recipes of nutritious foods made at home for babies as prepared by members of the Childbirth Education Association of Minneapolis/St. Paul.

Solve Your Child's Sleep Problems, by Richard Ferber, M.D. (New York: Simon & Schuster, 1985) is a useful and practical guide.

Index